T0193730

# The Lymphatic-Friendly DIET

## Kristin Osborn

**BALBOA**
PRESS

A DIVISION OF HAY HOUSE

Author Credits: Recipes by David Osborn

Balboa Press books may be ordered through booksellers or by contacting:

Balboa Press
A Division of Hay House
1663 Liberty Drive
Bloomington, IN 47403
www.balboapress.com.au
1 (877) 407-4847

Print information available on the last page.

ISBN: 978-1-5043-0358-3 (sc)
ISBN: 978-1-5043-0357-6 (e)

Balboa Press rev. date: 08/25/2016

# Contents

# Acknowledgements

I would like to acknowledge and thank my husband for supporting and assisting me while both writing and compiling the recipes for this book. He is a shy man and didn't really have a choice in whether he was going to compile recipes and test them or not. He always graciously supports my ideas. Without him, this book would not have happened.

While on this journey, I learned to cook and help in the kitchen, when it comes to meal times. Helping with the cooking makes me feel more contributory to this area of our home life and more of a team player. I find it a nice way to unwind from my day and give the dog some play time as well, because I kick the ball for her while attending the BBQ.

I also would like to thank my many patients whose valued input and constant questions compelled me to write this book. I hope you all like it, learn from it, and relate to the input in the following pages. Without my patients, this book would not have become a reality.

# Mission Statement

Our mission for this book is to educate readers on the basic fundamentals of the lymphatic system. The recipes are for everyone, not just those who suffer from a lymphatic condition or professionals who study lymphatics. Everyone has the right to know about the enormous amount of work the lymphatic system has to do in order to keep us functioning at an optimal level, for quality longevity.

This is not a diet but a "butterfly effect," a natural morphing of your lifestyle, which will constantly evolve with you at your own pace and not against, like many fad diets do. This is not how much weight you can lose in a certain period of time but a life education experience that your body will respond to and naturally lose unwanted fat at its own pace.

I treat people with these conditions and lecture on these topics here in Australia. I also suffer from them myself and wanted to share my story with others who are unable to attend my clinic.

# Introduction

As a lymphatic sufferer and therapist in the field of lymphology, I thought it was relevant to share with you how this book came about.

When I was growing up, I was always sick. I had blood disorders, where I would get volcano-like blisters on my inner top thighs, which needed bandaging so I wouldn't wee on them. I also had constant croup, nightly pains in my stomach (I remember my mother gently rubbing my stomach to ease the pain so I could go to sleep), severe chickenpox (both on the inside and outside of my body), whooping cough, hepatitis A, sinusitis, pleurisy, and measles to name a few. I'm sure there was more, but I can't recall them all. To say the least, I was a sickly child.

My family and I went on a vacation when I was nine; that vacation was a turning point in my life for me, because it was at that time that my family mentioned that I was starting to get "thunder thighs" and "hippo hips"; they said I looked like the hippo out of Disney's *Fantasia*. That started me to become conscious about my legs; I noticed that one of my grandmothers always wore long pants to cover her legs up. She had "bad" legs all her life with vein issues, leg ulcers, constant bruising, and pain. One of my aunties had the typical "tree trunk" legs, and so did a female cousin of mine. My other grandmother suffered with painful, aching legs and bad veins; she often had to lay down because of the bad aching in her legs. At this point in time, my mother was quite slim.

When I reached high school, I did start to notice that my thighs were larger than the other girls. I went to an all-girls high school, where I had a lot to compare with. Like most young females, I excessively dieted and exercised, not really knowing what I was doing. I did lose weight, but it was definitely the starting point of my rollercoaster ride with weight gain and loss through the next twenty-five years.

The summer when I was fifteen, I went swimming at the local swimming pool. I was wearing my first bikini and felt like I finally was beginning to fit in. I had religiously dieted and exercised, lost weight, and had the confidence to put a bikini on. That was short-lived when a boy yelled out to me that I had a big bum and legs, adding that I shouldn't wear a bikini. All of my inhibitions came flooding back immediately. This was a huge blow to my self-confidence regarding my legs. I stopped swimming, and I wore shorts or long pants all the time. I have never worn a bikini since.

I reached my early twenties, and my roommate, who was always fit and slim, asked me to go on a cruise holiday with her. I said yes and then began an excessive, eight-month routine of early morning workouts, late afternoon workouts, and all weekend workouts, compiled with a Jenny Craig program. I lost so much weight that the company asked me to do a TV commercial for them, and I later joined them as a weight loss consultant. This was short-lived because in order to build my clientele base, I had to recruit clients who had gone through the program and put their weight back on. This didn't sit right with my ethics and philosophy. If they followed the program correctly, why did they put their weight back on, plus more? Many of these clients were Life Members, which took them down the road of losing weight, gaining weight, losing weight, gaining weight; wasn't this pattern setting them up for constant failure?

*There must be something else!* I thought.

I put all my weight back on and some more, just like everyone else.

I got a job at the local a la carte restaurant down the road; it was an Italian restaurant, and they gave us dinner before our shift, so I worked in an office all day, and then I worked there Wednesday through Sunday (and sometimes double shifts on the weekend). I ate a lot of pizza, garlic bread, and chocolates. I piled on the weight once more.

Another friend asked me if I would like to go to Europe for a vacation. She was also small and petite, so off to the gym I went. I didn't quite lose the same amount of weight this time, but it wasn't too bad of an effort.

I came home from Europe a little heavier and started a new job with a major advertising company. It was a very stressful position, and the hours were long, but I didn't mind because I was single and had the time to put in. I got home late every evening and was tired, so the first thing I found to eat, I called "dinner," which was usually some sort of processed TV dinner and anything else that I could get my hands on that would fill me up. This wasn't a good idea, because I ballooned out to nearly a hundred kilograms.

I was also a smoker; I thought, *If I smoke, I won't eat as much, and this will keep my weight down.* I was just kidding myself.

I never learned to cook because when I was about sixteen, my parents and I moved out of our old house into a newly built home. My brother was living with his girlfriend at the time, so he never stayed in the new house. My parents had never owned a new home before, and my mum started to act quite strangely. In her mind, she had to keep everything like new, so we weren't allowed to sit on the lounge, eat at the dining room table, get any food or drink for ourselves, or use the shower. My dad could only use the outside toilet! I was yelled at for mucking up my bed after sleeping in it, so I did the only thing I could do: I moved out.

When their house was finally sold, eight years later, the oven, dining table, kitchen, and my brother's room were all still untouched and brand new.

Every single night, we ate out at very expensive restaurants because that was all there was available in our area. This became very boring and very "unspecial." I could pick anything I wanted off the menu, so my diet was not good. We bought our lunch during the day and usually skipped breakfast or had it at work, which was also purchased. My mother is still like this today, if not a little worse.

This is why my cooking skills were minimal, to say the least.

I was at the advertising company for nine years; halfway through, I met my husband, David. He was raised in a completely different, mostly normal environment. His mum and stepdad went away to stay in their caravan for up to six weeks at a time, and David was the only one left living at home, so he learnt to cook and care for himself.

I went to dinner at his house when we first met and ate so much food because I had forgotten how nice home-cooked food was. They all found it rather funny how much food I ate. Maybe in my mind, I felt it was like the Last Supper, so I had to fill up on good food before it ceased. Thank goodness it never did.

When it was my turn to have David around to my place for dinner, he walked in the door, and I whipped open the freezer door to expose a whole freezer full of frozen meals. I casually asked him which one he wanted, to his horror. He had never been fed any food like this and didn't know what it was, so I offered him my favourite one. I overcooked it in the microwave, like I tended to do, and he very politely sat and ate some of it. After a while, he announced that he would have to go; unbeknownst to me, he went home that night and cooked himself dinner. When his mum asked how the date went, he said that he must be in love because he had come to the conclusion that he would have to become the cook in the household. After we married and moved in together, that arrangement suited me perfectly fine.

As time went on, I became pregnant with our son, Ben. I left my hectic advertising job and retrained as a remedial therapist. During the pregnancy, it suddenly occurred to me that I was responsible for the health of the child growing inside of me. I grew a conscience and started to eat quite well. I craved fruit, something I had hardly eaten prior; maybe my unborn child was trying to tell me something in a subtle way. When Ben was born and I was on maternity leave, I took great pride and interest in cooking Ben's meals.

I worked from home to be able to watch my baby grow. I wanted to be there when he needed me; for the first time in my life I was extremely happy. My home business of remedial massage grew quickly. I started to notice patients coming to me with enlarged arms due to their treatments for breast cancer. In my remedial training, I had learned a little about treating these patients, but I felt there was much more to learn.

When I learn something, I have to know everything about it. I suppose I am a little OCD about learning. Off I went for the next ten years, learning about the lymphatic system: how it works, what happens when it all goes wrong, and how to treat it when it does go wrong.

Through my studies, I learned about lipoedema, a fat disorder that mostly affects women. All of the symptoms matched my legs. On further investigations and more study, I found out this was definitely what I had. All the literature that I had studied stated that diet and exercise would not work to assist in reducing the thighs and legs. *This can't be right*, I thought, so I started to experiment with myself. After different foods, exercise, compression, herbs, and massage techniques, I went from a hundred kilograms to sixty-nine. All of these things work, but I found the lymphatic-friendly diet made the biggest difference and quickest, longest-lasting results.

After studying about nutrition, raw foods, food cravings, and emotional eating, and knowing my husband is the cook in the family, I gave him a food brief for what foods are friendly to the lymphatic system. I asked him to write some recipes to fit the brief. Along the way of developing and test cooking the recipes, I unknowingly learnt to cook. I am involved with the cooking every night and find it most enjoyable and relaxing.

I have kept my weight steady over the last eight years. No more yo-yo dieting. What I did was a lifestyle change for the better. I found that I can eat large amounts of food and a good variety of foods and still keep my weight at an optimal level, without any harsh gym workouts. It is rare any of us in my family get sick. We haven't been sick for years; my lipoedema slightly reversed and is in a paused state.

I call what happened to me the Butterfly Process. It's one that I haven't finished and probably won't. It is a change in lifestyle and eating habits.

Changing and morphing. It won't take five minutes, and it doesn't need to because you have your whole life in front of you to try new ways of eating, cooking, textures, and flavours. You will need to let your body adjust when you start to eliminate some foods because just like an addict, you will go through withdrawal symptoms before your body returns back to its natural state. It is a bit like having a virus on your computer and taking the computer back to factory default to fix the problem. You will also start to notice that when you do eat some of the foods you have eliminated, your body won't tolerate them and will respond in an unfavourable way, with digestive issues, weight gain, hormonal changes, and strange symptoms.

It's a matter of simply knowing what foods work with the lymphatic system for optimal digestion and immunity, without compromising on portion size or taste. My family eats this food, every day. There are no separate meals in our house because someone's on a diet and they can only eat certain foods, or they can only have small amounts and watch everyone else eat large plates and then feel envious and hungry later on. Diets make people resentful. We all eat the same food and a good helping of it, too.

I don't diet, and I feel very free, so I wanted to share my journey with everyone. These foods are for anyone who has a lymphatic system (which is everyone); the recipes are easy to cook, and there aren't any ingredients that can't be found at your local supermarket or grocer.

My dream is that you learn from this book, enjoy the recipes, and begin your own morphing at your own pace. It would truly make me happy for you to learn about these foods and make your own recipes to share with others to suit your tastes and your family's lifestyle.

# PART 1

---

# Understanding the Lymphatic System

# Chapter 1

# History of the Lymphatic System and Why No One Seems to Know about It

Way back in the sixteenth and seventeenth centuries, there were many papers written about "a milky, white substance" found deep within the body. Lymph fluid is a milky, white substance when it is mixed with fat cells, but usually lymph fluid is a yellowish colour that you can see when you burst a blister or have a weeping wound.

These writings were documented in Ayurvedic (Indian) medicine, traditional Chinese medicine, and Greek and other European writings. The study of the lymphatic system never gained any momentum back then, because when they tried to extract the fluid for testing, the very small, fragile vessels would break. They became impatient with this and found an alternative: veins. Using the veins, they could extract blood and then study it under microscopes, which led to many discoveries. Thus, the study of the circulatory system came about, and most medicine and diagnostics are based around finding out what is in the blood.

Between the 1960s and 1980s, an Australian husband-wife team called Casley-Smith made ground-breaking work with the lymphatic system by using certain techniques to reduce swelling in the limbs. These are still taught today. They also started a lymphology association to assist in addressing these issues.

From the 1970s to 1990s, Dr. Vodder, a Denmark-born remedial therapist, brought lymphatic massage training to North America: first Canada and later the United States. His technique is the main technique still taught worldwide today.

In 1980, the Foldi Institute in Germany began research, treatment, and education of patients and professionals on the lymphatic system.

The lymphatic system is the largest system in the body and, as you read, has been skimmed over time and time again throughout history. No one really took any notice of its importance until the 1960s. You may well ask yourself, "Why don't I know anything about it?" or "Why doesn't my doctor know about it?" Well, that is a fairly easy question to answer.

You might only learn about the lymphatic system when or if it becomes "broken," and maybe not even then. I will cover this later.

If it does become "broken," there is no cure. It will remain that way for life.

There are no prescription medications that will assist in its functioning properly again, and there are only a few surgeries that will address chronic cases. There are some experimental surgeries being performed, but surgery generally creates more damage to the lymphatic system because of the effects of internal scarring.

This is where food and education for management begin.

As a lymphatic therapist, I treat patients with broken lymphatic systems and educate them on how to manage their condition, to the best of my knowledge and with the products that are available.

Management demands knowledge of anatomy, lymphatic aids such as compression garments and herbs, skin care, exercise, self-massage, and infection control. Travel and diet advice is also important, which should be provided by a specially trained lymphoedema therapist.

What I would like to see is education, beginning with this book, for stopping or deterring this system becoming broken in the first place. In some patients, this is unavoidable, but in the majority of people, it can be achieved with the right information and early intervention.

The lymphatic system has two main functions: waste removal and immune-system building.

## Waste Removal

The lymphatic system is similar to your average plumbing system. As a therapist, my aim is clearing out fluid from larger pipes, so when I start moving fluid from smaller pipes, it has someplace to go.

Let's begin with the circulation system.

The circulation system consists of your arteries, veins, and capillaries. The blood is pumped around your body by your heart under blood pressure, similar to a watch battery that makes the hands move and the watch tick.

Veins are parallel and have valves that open and shut to move the blood around and prevent backflow. When a valve becomes broken, the blood will backflow slightly. This is called a "varicose" vein.

When the blood is pumped out of the heart, it needs to be re-oxygenised and cleaned in order to keep the major organs working properly. Some of this fluid seeps into the area between cells. Because cells are round, there are gaps in between, and this is where this fluid goes. Then it is picked up by the lymphatic system.

The lymph collectors soak up the fluid like little mops and buckets and begin transporting the fluid to lymph vessels.

Lymph vessels act similar to veins. They have valves that open and close when the fluid builds up, which moves the fluid on. However, unlike the circulation system, lymph fluid is not moved around by the heart but by smooth muscle that is attached to the walls of the lymph vessels. The muscle contracts and expands from movement, and this pushes the fluid on to its next port of call. Movement and breathing move lymph fluid around your body, and just like a watch without a battery, if you are not wearing the watch and put it away in the cupboard, it ceases to tick. This is the same with the lymphatic system. If you cease to move, it will too. It stops working during surgery and when patients are in a coma. There are special mattresses for comatose patients to lie on so their lymph fluid moves.

Lymph vessels are similar to a spider web. They are approximately the same size and strong yet fragile. They sit just under the surface of the skin. This forms the superficial lymphatic system, and it covers you from the top of your head to the tips of your toes. It is this system that is mainly treated by a lymphatic therapist. Remember that whatever you put on your skin or in your mouth will find its way to the lymphatic system for screening and cleaning.

When the lymph fluid has been picked up by the lymph collectors, the little mops and buckets, and transported to the lymph vessels, it goes along specific pathways to lymph nodes. Lymph nodes look and filter like little kidneys.

There are approximately 600 to 1,500 lymph nodes in your body, and just because someone is bigger than another, it doesn't mean he has more lymph nodes. (A horse has fewer lymph nodes than a dog.) It is all based around when you were coming through the Pearly Gates and God was handing out lymph nodes as to how many you were given. It has just been discovered that the lymphatic system is individual to each person, just like a fingerprint is.

Lymph nodes sit at various locations in the body and can range in size from pinheads to olives, depending on their location. They are found behind the knees, in the groin, in the elbow, under the armpits, down the side of the neck, and underneath and along the clavicle bone; the majority are found in the deep abdominal area. The dirty fluid that consists of dust, hormones, pollutants, dead cells, cell debris (particularly from surgery), viruses, excess proteins, and heavy metals enters the lymph node, where it is cleaned and screened, then exits the other side to continue moving through lymph vessels onto the next station.

The items that cannot be cleaned and sent back out the other side need to be held in the germinal centre of the lymph node like a little vault. These items are cancer cells, heavy metals, and proteins.

After all the cleaning and screening has been done from each section, which happens between six and twenty times per minute—six times during rest and up to twenty times during exercise—the fluid is moved through to the deep lymphatic system.

The superficial lymphatic system drips into the deep lymphatic system, similar to water that seeps through rock in an underground cave, by way of the greater omentum.

The greater omentum sits across your stomach and can be stretched out to several meters long if removed. It concertinas up to fit in and contains many lymph nodes and vessels. The lymph fluid drains into the deep lymph nodes, which are located around the pelvis and lumbar area for women, leaving the birth canal free, and around the prostate and lumbar area for men. The dirty lymph fluid goes into a reservoir called the cisterna chyli, where it is expelled through the kidneys. The clean lymph fluid runs up the thoracic duct and dumps back into the circulatory system by way of the internal left jugular vein, where it begins its journey back around the major organs.

To make a comparison, I will talk about it like the plumbing system.

After we go to the toilet, we flush, which sends water into the bowl, pushing the waste through a number of smaller pipes to larger and larger pipes until it eventually ends up at the treatment works. The solid products are treated and dissolved and go back to the ocean. This is how the waste side works in the lymphatic system.

Just imagine your body is like the toilet system. If your toilet gets blocked, sometimes with tree roots or someone flushing something they shouldn't have, the waste has a difficult time getting through the pipes. (In our bodies, we call it constipation.) If the waste comes back out of the toilet, we call this reflux. If the waste generally has an unpleasant odour, this might be bad breath, heavily coloured or stinky urine, or body odour. If there is a pipe that could burst, this resembles bloating. If the waste seeps into the yard, this will be like having diarrhoea. If any of the toilet problems did happen to you, I'm quite sure you wouldn't just leave it. You would call a plumber because everyone wants a working toilet, right?

This should be the case with your body, too. It needs to be assessed in order to prevent more complications. In medicine, they only treat the symptoms; something to ease the constipation. Well, maybe there is something else causing the constipation. They may only treat the reflux; maybe there is something else causing the reflux. Most times body, breath, or urine odour isn't bought to anyone's attention to be addressed, and this would be the same with bloating; maybe a good burp will help fix that. You may need to look a little closer to what your body is trying to tell you.

If you are experiencing any or all of these symptoms, it is your body's way of saying your lymphatic system and digestive system are under pressure. You need to get to the bottom of the symptoms (excuse the pun), and I generally start with food.

If we have a poor diet, our system reacts, causing a whole host of digestive issues.

## Digestive Issues Checklist

- reflux
- colic
- bloating
- burping
- gas

- diarrhoea
- constipation
- extreme body odour
- darkened urine with odour
- bad breath
- coated tongue
- pimples

Ways of easing digestion is not only choosing the right foods for you but also what you put with the foods, where you eat the food, and when you eat the food.

Try to eat foods and drink fluids at room temperature, warm or hot; this prevents the stomach muscles going into spasm when something cold goes down and prevents mucus build-up.

You can add "warming foods" to salads like cracked black pepper, lemon juice, chili, cilantro, or coriander. Cinnamon, ginger, and cumin are warming spices and can be added to cold desserts to warm them up.

Try eating fruit prior to a meal, because the acids may help to break down foods. If you have issues eating bread, try toasting it.

Where you eat and when is important also. Eating regular, small meals (breakfast, morning tea, lunch, afternoon tea, dinner, and supper – no later than three hours prior to going to bed – keeps the digestive fire burning); it is equally important to sit in a comfortable, relaxing place, without the distraction of phones or computers while eating. Chew slowly, and notice the aroma, flavour, and texture of what you are eating or drinking.

Red meat can take up to forty-eight hours to digest and requires a large amount of water to break it down; this can clog digestion and lead to dehydration.

These are just some of the dietary issues connected with a poorly functioning lymphatic system; I will go further into this later on.

## Digestion and Lymphatic Waste Test

Eat corn kernels, medium diced capsicum, or passion fruit seeds, swallowing them whole, not chewing prior, and then see how quickly your digestion works by noticing when it comes out via the bowel. A good digestion would take approximately eight to twelve hours. It is not a quick digestion, when you need to go after twenty minutes of eating something; this means that it hasn't agreed with you.

If you take a vitamin supplement with a fluorescent in it, like Vitamin B, you can see how long it takes to work through your kidneys when you go to urinate; if you're not taking a supplement with a fluorescent, you can eat asparagus. This will work the same way, only notice the smell when you urinate. This will indicate how fast your lymphatic flow is. A good flow would be four hours to have clear or odour-free urine.

You can also see how long the colour or smell stays around; this will indicate how hydrated you are, urine should be as clear as possible, the more yellow-brown your urine is would indicate that you are very dehydrated.

Most people I encounter are dehydrated due to one reason or another; they may not drink enough water, they may be on fluid tablets, or they may eat foods that are high in salt. When these people try to start drinking water, it is usually short-lived because they get fed up with going to the toilet and urinating all the time. I'd like you to think of it in another way. If you have a potted plant and don't water it for many months, you will notice the soil shrinking away from the sides of the pot. If you try to water the plant, the water will simply run off. What needs to be done is to sit the plant in a basin of water for it to slowly absorb the water and become saturated again. If you start by drinking a cup of water after you have had a coffee or tea, you will start to slowly increase your fluid amount each day. You can gradually add a cup of water to your midmorning snack, lunch, afternoon snack, and dinner, and you will have increased your fluid intake slowly. If you do go to the toilet more frequently, I find this will start to subside after approximately three weeks, when your cells have started to uptake the fluid.

Hydration helps with detoxifying through urination and regular bowel movements, and it may assist with regulating body temperature. Hydration doesn't just come from water or drinks; it can come from the following foods:

apples
bananas
blueberries
broccoli
broth
cabbage
capsicums
carrots
cauliflower
celery
cucumbers
eggplant
grapes
lettuce
melons
mushrooms
oranges
peaches
pineapples
plums
strawberries
tomatoes
yoghurt
water ice blocks made with fruit

This is your waste removal side of the lymphatic system; next we will look at the immunity side.

# No. 2 Immune Building

If we get injured or sick, it is our lymphatic system that comes to the rescue. I like to think of it like a knight in shining armour.

These knights in shining armour are called white blood cells and killer T-cells.

In order to produce these cells, we have lymphoid organs to help out. Our bodies have approximately three litres of lymph fluid; the fluid contains white blood cells and is made in our first lymphoid organ, bone marrow. It then seeps into the area between the cells, where it is picked up by the lymph collectors, the little mops and buckets, and released into the lymphatic system for distribution.

The cells are then stored in these lymphoid organs, ready for when invaders come in to attack our system and cause us problems. White blood cells and killer T cells act similarly to Pac-man, gobbling up the invaders trying to destroy us. Lymphoid organs include bone marrow, tonsils, thymus, spleen, Peyer's patches and appendix.

## Bone Marrow

Produces red blood cells and platelets for the circulatory system and white blood cells, which are the basis of lymph fluid. This fluid is the crucial component in fighting off foreign invaders coming into the body and supporting the body's health.

You can see what lymph fluid looks like when you have a blister and burst it. The yellow sticky fluid which flows out is lymph fluid.

## Tonsils

These lymphoid organs are the first point of contact for any viruses trying to enter through the nose or the mouth. They will become sore, red, and inflamed, alerting you to fix this problem before the virus goes further into the body. In the old days, surgeons used to take them out because they didn't have an understanding of how important they are. Nowadays, they have a little more understanding and are not as quick to schedule their removal. However, due to the superbugs we have around today, the tonsils can't fight viruses off like they used to.

If you happen to get tonsillitis a lot, I would first start to gargle with a chemist-prepared antibacterial or good old-fashioned salt and warm water; step up your oral hygiene by drinking lots of water, brushing your teeth after each meal, and regular flossing. When I know of a teen who suffers from many bouts of tonsillitis, I often ask them if they have been kissing a lot and how good their oral hygiene is. They usually blush, but I know this is generally the problem. If you do continue to get tonsillitis, and you have followed these tips, then a trip to the doctor is recommended.

## Thymus

This lymphoid organ is our second line of defense.

The thymus is located in front of the heart and behind the sternum and looks similar to a thick sausage that has been bent in half.

This lymphoid organ is the factory centre for killer T cells. These are a type of white blood cell that can kill cancer cells, foreign invader cells, or damaged cells.

The thymus is most active from birth to twelve years; this is the time when killer T cells are produced. After that time, the thymus shrinks and turns into a fat lump. This is crucial information to know, and we need to make sure that our children have the best diet possible to produce as many of these killer T cells before it shrinks and turns to fat. The amount of killer T cells they make will need to defend their system for the rest of their life, and with many new strains of super viruses in the world today, we need to get serious with what we are feeding the next generation.

## Spleen

The spleen is located on the left side of the body, above the stomach and under the ribs. It is the largest lymphoid organ. The spleen acts like a large lymph node, cleaning, screening, and filtering blood. It keeps body fluids balanced, creates white blood cells, stores red blood cells and blood platelets.

When you have a foreign invader, the spleen sends out immune cells to fight it off and keep us healthy, similar to an army that is deployed to attack and save the castle.

## Peyer's Patches

These lymphoid nodules are named after their founder and located in the small intestine and ileum. We have approximately fifteen to twenty-five nodes, and like the thymus, these nodes decline coming into adulthood.

Peyer's patches clean and screen everything in the small intestine. When they don't function properly, it is commonly called leaky gut or sticky gut syndrome. The patient may experience symptoms of reflux, colic, bloating, burping, irritable bowel, constipation, and diarrhoea, to name a few.

When you look at a healthy gut with Peyer's patches, you can see a smooth outer lining of the intestines and many lymph nodes, along with killer T cells patrolling along the line, looking out for any bad bacteria that wants to enter, but when you have Peyer's patches syndrome, the outer lining of the intestines is rough, there are not many lymph nodes or killer T cells, and there are spaces open to let bad bacteria through. Once again, diet assists with healing this condition.

## Appendix

The appendix is located near the right hip bone and aids in the removal of waste from the digestive system.

It stores good bacteria and can repopulate the digestive tract after a bout of diarrhoea.

There is not much information about the appendix because most medical people believe it is something left behind after evolution, but it has been included as a lymphoid organ, and I like to think that we have been given everything in our body that we need for one purpose or another; it wouldn't have been created for no reason.

Lymph vessels run through the liver; this assists with regenerating and repairing the liver after it has been damaged. Lymph vessels have been found recently in the brain; the best way to drain them to date is through deep breathing exercises.

# When It All Goes Wrong

## Lymphoedema

"Lymphoedema" means "oedema" or swelling of the lymphatic system.

Lymphoedema is the name given to the problem associated with a broken lymphatic system.

There are two types of lymphoedema. Lymphoedema may occur straight away or develop years later.

## Primary Lymphoedema

Some people are born with a broken lymphatic system. It's a bit like "Goldilocks and the Three Bears," as I will explain next.

1.  Patients will be born with not enough lymph vessels, or they can be too small to accommodate the amount of lymph fluid needed to pass through.

2. Patients will be born with lymph vessels that are too large, allowing too much fluid to pass through, causing a back-up effect or "traffic jam."

3. Patients will be born with an absence of lymph collectors, lymph nodes, or capillaries, or the lymph nodes are fibrous and won't allow adequate lymph fluid to pass through.

Primary lymphoedema can be diagnosed at birth; the baby usually presents with an enlarged foot. However, some people don't develop primary lymphoedema for some time, in their teens or after the age of thirty-five. Patients can have both primary and secondary lymphoedema at the same time.

**Secondary Lymphoedema**

Patients are born with a fully functioning lymphatic system, but something goes wrong and lymph vessels become compromised or lymph nodes are removed. This is the type of lymphoedema most people will know about.

**Causes of Secondary Lymphoedema**

- cancer treatments, both surgical (the removal of lymph nodes) and radiation (which destroys lymph vessels)
- scar tissue formed from surgeries, particularly cancer, abdominal surgery, and knee replacements
- needles or blood pressure cuffs used on a limb that has had lymph nodes removed, has been radiated, or has a large amount of scarring
- burns
- multiple sprains and strains, which cause tissue scarring, particularly in ankles
- heat combined with obesity
- immobility and lack of movement
- obesity
- insect bites
- dog or cat scratches on an affected limb
- recurrent infections
- leg ulcerations

- vein problems
- restrictive clothing, including tight jeans, shoes, socks, jewellery, improperly fitted compression garments
- plane travel
- a fall on an affected limb
- other medical factors: congenital heart failure; kidney problems; thyroid, liver, or lung problems

In secondary lymphoedema, the lymph fluid still fills the spaces, but it has a difficult time getting back through; it wants to keep moving, but an obstruction (damaged lymph vessels or built-up scar tissue) or a dead end (removed lymph nodes) has occurred.

Similar to driving along the freeway doing 100 KMH and suddenly there are road works ahead, all lanes must merge into one and the speed limit is reduced to 40 KMH. This creates a backup of fluid, or traffic jam, or the fluid just meets a dead end, preventing lymph flow.

Secondary lymphoedema can happen from the tip of the head to the toes. You may know of someone having an arm or leg that's larger than the other or swollen feet, but patients can also have swelling in both limbs, all limbs, the face, the neck, the abdomen, the genitals, or the whole body. This can depend on the severity of their cancer treatment, multiple surgeries, obesity, or an underlying fat disorder.

## Lymphoedema Checklist

- oedema or swelling in the limb, head, neck, abdomen, or genitals
- pain in the affected area
- weight gain
- fatigue
- a sense of tightness in the affected area
- tingling or pins and needles in the affected area
- aching limbs and joints
- a sense of heaviness in the affected area

- reduced function or limited range of movement in the effected limb
- sleeping difficulties
- psychological distress
- poor body image, coupled with depression
- social and sexual isolation

A special thank you for the patients who participated in lending the following photos.

Unilateral arm swelling caused by breast cancer

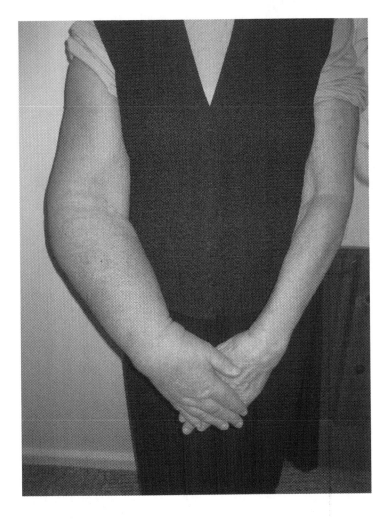

Unilateral leg swelling caused by ovarian cancer and
bilateral feet swelling caused by diabetes

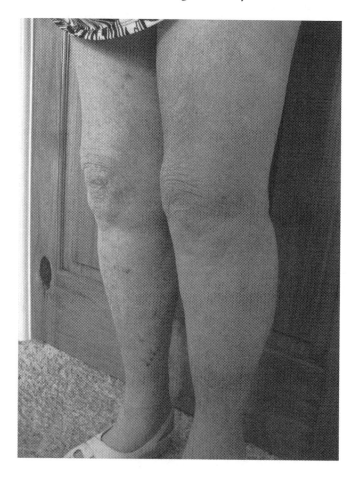

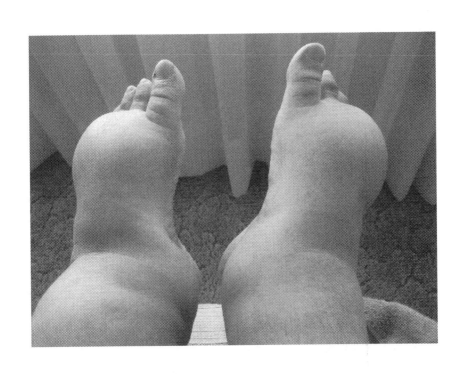

# Lipoedema

Lipoedema is one of those underlying fat disorders which can cause unexplained swelling; this is the condition that I suffer from.

Lipoedema is a genetic disorder which mainly affects females with a white European background; males can also have it, but it is much harder to diagnose. It is rare in people of Asian background.

Patients who suffer from lipoedema have generally a fully functioning lymphatic system until it becomes broken.

It becomes broken due to various problems, including obesity (stage 3), vein issues, inflammation, scarring from surgeries, hormonal imbalances, thyroid problems, and changes in steroid levels from chemotherapy, to name a few. Patients can get swelling in the feet; this then becomes known as lipo-lymphoedema. Fat tissue is constantly leeching hormones and inflammatory markers. Now the lymphatic system is broken.

# Lipoedema Checklist

- it occurs from people with anorexia to the morbidly obese.
- it occurs bilaterally (both legs) and symmetrically from the waist to the ankles
- lipoedema fat cannot be lost through excessive diet or excessive exercise; this often can make the condition worse.
- the disease is usually triggered around the hormonal changes at puberty, pregnancy, pre-menopause, or post-menopause, and following gynaecological surgery due to changes in oestrogen.
- patients will gain weight in lipoedema areas (around the hips, thighs, upper arms, and abdomen) and lose it in non-lipoedema areas (face and breasts).
- the basic profile of a sufferer looks like a size 8 from the waist up and a size 16 from the waist down.
- patients can have column or tree trunk-looking legs.

- patients can have flat feet or inverted or knocked knees; this can lead to knee or hip replacements later on.
- digestive issues, including Gastroesophageal reflux disease and Irritable bowel syndrome are common inflammatory diseases: arthritis, osteoarthritis, fibromyalgia and gout are common
- patients can have an auto-immune disease: sjogren's, reynaud's, or lupus.
- lordosis: dipping in the lower back.
- hyper mobile joints, being overly flexible.
- low elasticity or marshmallow-like skin surface (e.g., cellulite).
- pain and heaviness in the legs.
- patients will easily bruise due to weak vein walls.
- cold skin temperature in the lower extremities
- spider or varicose veins.
- bloating.
- the need to get up multiple times a night to urinate.
- difficulty sleeping.
- poor concentration.
- patients may weigh more at night.
- heart palpitations.
- hair loss.
- shortness of breath.

If you have some of these symptoms, you need to get it properly diagnosed to start on a lymphatic program. I run a program for this in Australia.

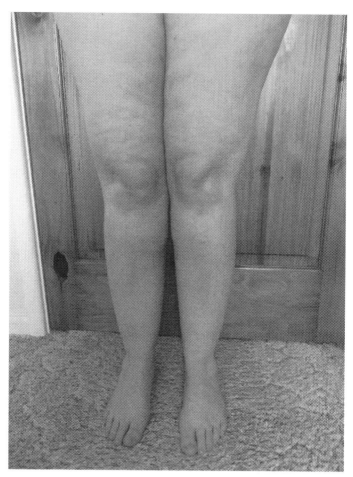

Stage 1-2

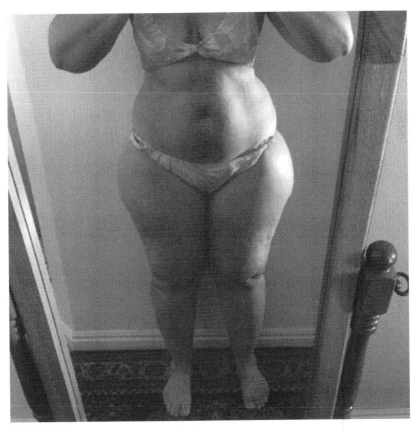

Stage 2-3

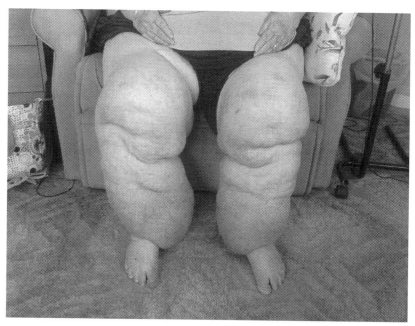

Stage 4

# PART 2

---

# The Lymphatic Way

I was bewildered to see how many food pyramids are out there, from the downright crazy to the extreme of cutting out certain food groups. Balance of all food groups is the key, unless you have an intolerance and need to cut out certain items, but you should always have the education to know what to replace that group with, so you don't miss out on vital nutrients.

I was watching a UK documentary called *The World's Best Diet.* The movies ranked countries and Adventists are ranked as well according to their food intake. I noticed some interesting information that came through:

Iceland is No. 1, due to geothermal cooking; they make a rye bread that is extremely high in fibre, and their diet is high in fish, with very little processed foods.

Italy is No. 2, due to small towns growing organic food and meat and making absolutely everything themselves. People living in smaller regions have little access to processed foods.

Greece is No. 3, due to their Mediterranean diet.

Seventh Day Adventists are No. 4, due to their vegetarian/vegan diet. People following a vegan diet have a life expectancy of approximately seven years longer than the average person, and people following a vegetarian diet have a life expectancy of approximately five years longer than the average person. Food for thought.

Japan is No. 5, due to their high fish, seafood, and broth meals.

If you have a look at the top five diets, they eat more fish, seafood, organic fruit, and vegetables, and they consume very little meat (if any meat at all).

Some food pyramids suggest eating like they did in the caveman days, largely meat and meat products. That was a time when everything was truly organic and soils were virgin soils; there was no acid rain, no pesticides, no dropped nuclear bombs, no germ warfare, no contaminated water supplies and no air pollutants. Animals, including fish, weren't pellet fed with added growth hormones and antibiotics, living in sheds. Everything was in abundance, and people had all day to find food. This type of eating is simply not practical for the lives that we are living today.

Let's fast forward to modern day living. We need to learn food skills for fighting the food challenges we face today, which are our modern-day dinosaurs.

Food companies put chemicals in our foods and spray chemically made vitamins on our food so they can say it has vitamins and minerals, to make bigger profits. There is a labyrinth of food labels and genetically modified foods. Supermarkets and marketing companies tell us what to buy and when, for their profit not our health. We are bombarded with advertising, catalogues, and all forms of media, showing happy times and gaining friends by consuming processed foods that are high in saturated fats and sugars.

All of our soils, air, water, and oceans are now polluted, and we are time poor. Our bodies do adapt to a certain degree, but we are certainly pushing the boundaries and seeing the effects.

We are seeing more diseases, allergies, cancers, autoimmune disorders, and obesity, which comes with other complications. Our lymphatic system is telling us, quite loudly, that something needs to change and there is no time to spare, particularly for our children and their future.

I have put together the Lymphatic-Friendly Food Pyramid, which I believe represents a combination of all the good food pyramids put together.

It is a generalised food pyramid and does not encompass any specific dietary conditions like celiac, salicylate, or lactose-intolerant, and so on. Please use your own discretion or consult a dietician for any specific dietary needs.

## Lymphatic-Friendly Food Pyramid

Try to avoid alcohol, caffeine, processed and packaged foods, UHT milk, refined sugars, and all white sugar, pasta, flour, and breads. Increase organics where possible, and look for foods that have a short list of ingredients (or none at all): fresh fruit and vegetables. Use the KISS rule: Keep It Simple and Sensible. Eat a variety of coloured, fresh foods daily with plenty of fluids, keeping the not-so-good foods to a minimum.

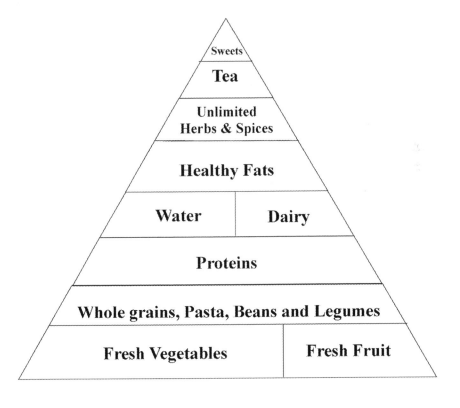

# Food Pyramid Breakdown

## Supplements

Supplements are only necessary to balance any holes in your diet.

A good quality multivitamin along with calcium and Vitamin D (because most people don't get enough sunlight), taken daily, are very good basic supplements to add.

## Sweets

Sweets are necessary to provide balance. Fruit in any capacity is a good sweetener to reduce sugar cravings and increase fibre, hydration, and vitamin intake. These are just a few suggestions.

1 piece or square of 85 percent dark chocolate; can be whole or grated and placed on top of fruit

1 scoop of fruit sorbet in a wafer (not waffle) cone

2 plain biscuits

1 homemade piece of plain cake (no icing or cream)

2 plain pikelets

1 crêpe filled with fresh fruit

## Tea

2-3 cups green, white, oolong, black, or herbal (caffeine-free) tea per day.

Tea provides good antioxidants and is known for aiding good digestion, reducing bad cholesterol, and avoiding heart ailments. It is used as a preventative for breast cancer and can also provide relief from asthma.

## Herbs and Spices

Are used unlimited, they add amazing depth of flavour and really brings drab food to life, as well as the health benefits that go along with them. They may be used fresh, dried, powdered, frozen, steeped to make a tea or added to milk or smoothies.

### Healthy Fats

These are necessary to regulate metabolism and should not be skipped to save on calories. Take 3-7 servings per day.

1 teaspoon olive oil

1 teaspoon coconut oil

1 teaspoon flax seed oil,

1 teaspoon MCT oil (used in salad dressings or sauces for cooking but not frying)

30 grams avocado

3 walnuts or almonds

## Water

A *minimum* of 8 cups/250 millilitres of plain, mineral, or soda water (containing no sulphites; you will need to check the label for these), preferably with lemon, daily.

If you drink coffee, after finishing your cup, refill it with water and drink it; this will counterbalance the effects of the coffee. Remember to check your urine to make sure it is clear; if not, this indicates the need for more water.

## Dairy

Some people have problems digesting traditional dairy, as I do, so I limit my intake but replace the calcium I am not getting with traditional dairy products with plant-based calcium to make sure I have met my dietary needs.

Most people don't have a problem with traditional dairy products; this is a general daily guideline:

1 glass/250 millilitres of milk (almond milk can also be used) in tea, coffee, smoothies, or sauces.

40 grams of cheese (feta, mozzarella, or parmesan); this can be used in salads, on hamburgers or sandwiches, grated over pizza or oven bakes, or in soups and sauces.

200 grams of natural yoghurt (not Greek); this can be placed on top of casseroles, spaghetti, or Mexican dishes; used in smoothies; or flavoured with fruit for dessert.

## Proteins

70 grams lean red meat or pork (preferably organic and pulled), twice a week.

These types of meats take longer to break down and digest, requiring more water, which can make you dehydrated; they also cause inflammation. I personally don't eat them but know some diehard carnivores, so you will find it used in some of the recipes in this book. At the bottom of these recipes, David has provided a substitute protein.

Up to six eggs per week (preferably organic or free range).

5 200 gram servings of chicken (preferably organic or free range) or wild-caught fish per week.

Particularly oily fish like Atlantic salmon and sardines. Other fish types are cod, haddock, plaice, and herring, not excluding tinned tuna, salmon, and kippers in spring water (trans fat free).

The key to look for is "wild caught." Other seafood varieties include oysters, prawns, and calamari.

½ cup firm tofu

## Whole Grains, Pasta, Legumes

Up to 5-7 servings per day consisting of:

½ cup cooked brown rice, wild rice, farro, barley, quinoa, oats, whole meal or spelt pasta, whole meal cous cous, rice or buckwheat noodles, chick peas, black beans, red kidney beans, mixed beans, split peas, or lentils.

1 slice seeded, wholegrain, soy, or linseed bread.

## Vegetables

Up to 7 servings per day, with unlimited leafy greens. Vegetables should consist of all different colours; generally limit any vegetable that is white or starchy. Vegetables can be eaten raw, cooked, or whole juiced.

# Fruit

3 servings per day, either whole or chopped. Fruit can be eaten raw, dried, cooked, or whole juiced. Try to eat different colours.

## My 7-Day Eating Guide

Many patients ask me what I eat and when; the following is how I put my food pyramid together. This is only a guideline of what I do.

It looks a like this:

### Before Breakfast, 5.30 a.m.

Juice of ½ lemon or 2 lemon cubes in a cup of hot water + another cup of plain water.

### Breakfast, 7.00 a.m.

### During the Week

2 Weet-Bix or breakfast biscuits with 50 ml milk + 75 ml water and 1 banana, or ½ cup whole oats with ¼ cup milk + ½ cup water and 1 banana, or 1 cup breakfast Muesli with yoghurt (recipe in this book).

### Weekends

2 pieces of whole grain toast with 1 poached egg and ½ cup beans or 1 piece of fruit toast with organic butter.

### Morning Tea, 8.30 a.m. - 10.00 a.m.

1 cup caffeine-free tea with either guacamole, hummus, or salsa (all recipes in this book) on 4 water crackers, or 2 dried dates and a cup of water.

## Lunch, 12.00 p.m. - 1.30 p.m.

### During the Week

2 sandwiches on wholegrain bread with salad and either fish, chicken, cheese, or egg. 2 cups of water and 1 piece of fruit; I sneak in a piece of 85 percent dark chocolate.

### Weekends

2 cups of water, a large bowl of fresh salad with fish, and lentil or vegetable soup or chicken soup with lentils, and a piece of fruit.

## Afternoon Tea, 3.30 p.m.

1 cup caffeine-free tea and a cup of water with trail mix (almonds or walnuts and a piece of raw coconut; recipe in this book) or a piece of fruit.

## Dinner, 6.00 p.m.

### During the Week

1 cup water, at least 5 vegetables, and 2 servings of whole grains, pasta, or legumes with either chicken or fish (I don't eat red meat or pork).

### Weekends

Pizza (vegetarian on flatbread), pasta, vegetable omelettes/frittatas, or open sandwiches (all recipes in this book).

## After Dinner, 7.00 pm

1 cup green tea + 1 cup of water with either:

1 fruit-filled crepe

2 scoops banana gelato

1 small bowl baked fruit salad

1 poached pear

1 piece of date and walnut cake

1 scoop fruit sorbet in a wafer cone

## Food Keys

In the following recipes, you will notice these symbols next to each food ingredient: **ai, al, ac, p,** and **mct.**

Some foods may have only one symbol, while others have multiple symbols. The reason behind this is to get to know types of foods and important principles of that food type that contain properties which help assist the lymphatic system. This will also help to educate you to make better food ingredient choices.

**ai** = anti-inflammatory foods

**al** = alkalising foods

**ac** = acid-forming foods

**p** = potassium-rich foods

**mct** = foods containing medium chain triglycerides (healthy fats)

Anti-inflammatory foods assist in getting rid of inflammation caused by other foods, mostly processed and packaged foods.

Inflammation in the body causes or exacerbates many problematic conditions.

- Arthritis
- Osteoarthritis
- Rheumatoid arthritis
- Fibromyalgia
- Gout
- Lymphoedema
- Lipoedema
- Lupus
- Asthma
- Pleurisy
- Eczema
- Dermatitis
- Psoriasis
- Gastritis
- Sinusitis
- Hepatitis
- Vasculitis
- Chrohn's disease
- Colitis
- Diverticulitis
- Skin disorders
- Irritable Bowel
- Cancer
- Hay Fever
- Periodontitis
- Obesity
- Heart Disease

It is vital to know what foods can work the opposite to start to calm the system down.

It's not only processed or packaged foods which can cause inflammation; when you eat too much of a certain food group, your body gets an overload and sees it as an invader; you will become inflamed.

Ever since my son, Ben, was a baby, he was a huge milk drinker; he hardly touched water, but I thought it was a healthier option than fizzy drinks or fruit juices, which are high in sugar, so I let him drink his milk. In winter time, he always developed croup and was put on heavy steroids and asthma puffers. I never looked forward to this time of year, as I knew I would be cleaning up mucous vomit or rushing him to the hospital in the middle of the night because he was turning blue from not being able to breathe.

I had him breathing in the steam from the shower, we had vaporisers on in his room, he would go on antibiotics constantly; it was a mystery to the medical profession why he was still getting croup at the age of ten, when children should grow out of it by three.

One afternoon, while drinking his milk, he began scratching and scratching and complaining about a rash he had developed. I told him for the next seven days, he was to leave out all dairy from his diet and try to reboot his system. He did this, but quite reluctantly, because when he left out the dairy, he had to start to drink water. After seven days, I reintroduced milk at one cup per day only but kept the water; from that day onwards, he has never had croup or mucous vomit or needed steroids, antibiotics, or puffers.

He now has his milk, yoghurt, and cheese but only the amount he requires for his diet, with plenty of water in between.

The starting key to help reduce inflammation is food.

**Examples of Anti-inflammatory Foods**

leafy greens and kale
wild-caught oily fish, salmon and sardines
fish supplements
kelp and nori sheets
spirulina

garlic and ginger
fruit particularly papaya
beans and legumes
raw nuts, walnuts and seeds
herbal, oolong, green and white tea
sweet potato
brussel sprouts
cauliflower
fennel
herbs and spices
broccoli and red cabbage
hemp and chia seeds
tofu
celery
cacao
beets
turmeric and saffron
extra virgin olive oil
avocados
cranberries and blueberries
asian mushrooms

Acid and alkalising foods are both necessary for a balanced diet; you will find a balance in all of our recipes.

A pH of 7.0 is neutral for your blood. Below this number means that you have too much acid in your blood, and above this number means you have too much alkaline in your blood. Blood should be slightly alkaline at about 7.35-7.45. You can get test kits to find out your pH levels, either through your urine or saliva.

Acid blood can come from acid-forming foods, stress, toxicity, or depriving the cells of oxygen and other nutrients. The body will try to compensate by finding alkaline minerals, but if the diet doesn't contain enough, a build-up of acids will lead to disease.

High acid decreases the body's ability to absorb minerals and nutrients; it also decreases cell energy production, cell repair, and removal of heavy metals. Tumour cells thrive with acid, making you feel fatigued and susceptible to illness.

For health restoration, the diet should consist of 80 percent alkaline and 20 percent acid foods, and to maintain health, it should be 60 percent alkaline and 40 percent acid.

## Examples of Extremely Alkaline Foods

lemons
watermelon
baking soda

It may seem that citrus foods are high acid, but when they are digested, the body converts them into an alkaline.

## Examples of Neutral Foods

organic butter
distilled water
plain natural yoghurt

## Examples of Alkalising Foods

most fresh fruit and vegetables
herbs and spices
mineral water
organic soy milk
tofu
almonds
chestnuts
apple cider vinegar
some alkalising minerals: calcium, magnesium and potassium.

## Examples of Calcium-Rich Foods (other than Dairy)

broccoli
almonds
collards
bok choy
pumpkin seeds
okra
leeks
artichokes
avocado
celery
green beans
raw coconut
onions
fennel
Swiss chard
butternut pumpkin
kale
spinach
Brussel sprouts
mulberries
cabbage
asparagus
raw sesame seeds
navel oranges
wild-caught salmon
sardines
black-eyed peas
potato
fish with edible bones

## Examples of Magnesium-Rich Foods

raw sesame seeds
dill
basil
broccoli
almonds
okra
flaxseeds
spinach
chives
chard
black beans
plain natural yoghurt
avocado
85 percent dark chocolate

## Examples of Potassium-Rich Foods

white beans
leafy greens
plain natural yoghurt
salmon
snapper
cod
tuna
whiting
perch
bream
sardines
prawns
pork
minced beef
lamb
bacon
avocado

mushrooms

bananas

nectarines

pineapples

mangoes

dried dates

almonds

baked beans

homemade soup

potatoes (with skin on or mashed)

spinach

fennel

sweet potato

tomatoes

pumpkins

parsnips

We need potassium-rich foods because they remove the salt and built-up proteins, which can cause infection, out of our system.

## Examples of Acid-Forming Foods

corn

lentils

blueberries

cranberries

currants

plums and prunes

canned, dried (except dates), or glazed fruits

most grains, beans, and legumes

dairy

animal protein

artificial sweeteners

energy drinks

coffee

medications

alcohol
refined white grains
processed foods
processed soy products
fried foods
fast foods

Soft drinks are acidic and contain phosphoric acid, which leaches magnesium out of the body, causing cramping and decreasing bone density.

## Medium Chain Triglycerides (Healthy Fats)

MCTs are easily metabolised due to their solubility in water, which means they can be absorbed at a higher rate; they do not need bile salts to be digested and are less likely to be stored in our fat cells. They have been shown to help burn excess calories, causing weight loss.

Longer chain fats are absorbed through the lymphatic system, causing strain.

Because MCTs don't require energy for absorption, use, or storage, people with malnutrition and malabsorption problems or cancer can benefit by eating these types of food.

### Examples of Medium Chain Triglyceride-Type Foods

coconut oil
olive oil
MCT oil
avocados
almonds
walnuts
85 percent dark chocolate

## Long Chain Triglycerides

These are absorbed through the lymphatic system, making it digest rather than build immunity and remove waste, its main function.

### Examples of These Foods

Saturated fats from animal products; processed meats such as salami, sausages, and ham; tasty cheese; cream cheese; lard; butter; whipping cream; mayonnaise; and duck fat.

## Anthocyanins: Purple Fruit and Vegetables

There has been recent information coming out of the breeding program at the Applethorpe Research Station, run by Bruce Topp and Dougal Russell, regarding the Queen Garnet Plum. They found that it had very high levels of anthocyanins, an antioxidant linked to numerous positive health benefits.

Scientists have been surprised by the plum's health benefits.

"When we first started working with some of these types of compounds no one believed something as simple as a plum could actually be a medicine," Professor Lindsay Brown, from the University of Southern Queensland in Toowoomba, said.

He said it was not surprising there was global interest in the fruit after he was astonished by the results of a trial he oversaw last year.

"We gave plum juice to obese rats with the same health problems humans have from being overweight," Professor Brown said.

"They had high blood pressure, a fatty liver, poor heart function and arthritis.

"When we put the plum juice in their food it all came back to normal without changing their diet."

They lost weight, while their blood pressure, fat levels, as well as liver and heart function all returned to normal levels.

*Information courtesy of Landline ABC News*

Anthocyanins are antioxidant compounds and are a polyphenol subclass responsible for the dark colouring in many fruit and vegetables. Anthocyanins also provide the food industry with nonsynthetic food colourings.

There is a large and increasing worldwide bank of research evaluating the health benefits of antioxidants and anthocyanins; this has been summarised by Ghosh and Konishi at the *"Combined fruit industry conference 2013 with The Good Rich Food Company"* into the following list:

antioxidant
anti-allergic
anti-inflammatory
anti-viral
anti-proliferative
anti-mutagenic
anti-microbial
anti-carcinogenic
cardiovascular protective
microcirculation improvement
diabetes improvement

**Foods Containing Anthocyanins**

queen garnet plum (the highest)
plums
eggplant
black currants
purple asparagus

cranberries
blueberries
blackberries
mulberries
chokeberries
acai berries
red cabbage
red and purple grapes
kidney beans
black beans
pomegranates
red fleshed peaches
red fleshed oranges
cherries
red and purple olives
purple carrots
purple potatoes
purple sweet potato
purple string beans
purple snap peas
red onion
purple kale
purple lettuce
beetroot
purple tomatoes
bananas

## Foods to Avoid

## Sulphates (Mineral Salts) and Preservatives

Some people experience digestive problems or allergies connected with sulphates, mineral salts, and preservatives found in foods. Some food packaging may list these by name or number or not at all, so it is vital, particularly if you have a severe allergy, to read labels and steer away from food products that are known to set you off. This can be difficult, however.

I had a bad experience on my last holiday. My husband and I thought it would be a good idea to get some fresh prawns, from the local fish co-op, for lunch. David usually does all the peeling because I am too slow, and he usually sneaks a prawn or two when peeling, but this particular day he didn't.

We started to eat, and I made a comment on how salty the prawns were. I asked if he had added any salt because I don't use salt, but he said he hadn't. He also commented on how unusually salty the prawns were. I thought, *I am going to have to drink more water today to counteract the salt.* David likes to eat the heads of the prawns, and he said they were even saltier than the prawns.

Within approximately thirty minutes, I started to scratch my upper chest area and thought I must have been bitten by something. The rash became hot and flared across my whole chest and up my neck. I always carry a four-way action cream with me which consists of an antiseptic, antihistamine, anaesthetic, and anti-inflammatory, so I put that on along with a cold pack. That seemed to sooth it; still, it didn't cross my mind that I was having an allergic reaction.

That night, I was going to bed and asked David if he was coming too; he said he would be in shortly. Our room was quite light, so I could see quite easily, even without a light on. I rolled over and saw a very large black spider on David's pillow case. I have arachnophobia, so I jumped up and watched this spider crawl across his side of the bed and down. I screamed out to him, and he came running. I couldn't quite get my words out properly: "There's a, huh, huh, big, huh, huh, over there, this big, black spider!"

He just stood and looked at me. I remember thinking, *Why isn't he going over there and getting that spider?*

To my surprise, he said, "Darl, you're dreaming."

What? He grabbed my shoulders, steered me to the mirror, and said, "Look at your eyes; you're dreaming."

I looked into the mirror and did not recognise the person looking back at me. My eyes were as wide as saucers, and my pupils were dilated. I was having a night terror. I didn't believe him, so he ripped off all the sheets, picked up both mattresses, and put them up against the wall. He turned all the tables upside down to show me there was no spider in the room. I was still not convinced.

We remade the bed and fixed up the room and got into bed. I lay there fully dressed, scanning the room all night for that spider. I didn't sleep a wink.

In the morning, I was very tired and quite embarrassed by the night's antics. I could not work out why that incident had happened. David said he did. He is very observant. He said when we were at the fish co-op, he had noticed the prawns looked dull and dry. All of the fish in the window were filleted; there were no whole fish, and the green prawns were sold with their heads removed. He suggested the fish co-op didn't have a very high turnover rate of produce, and they used mineral salt to preserve it and make it last longer. We returned to the fish co-op that day, and they did admit they used mineral salt for that very reason.

I have never had such a severe allergic reaction to mineral salt before, and now when I go to buy "fresh" seafood, I ask if they have put any mineral salt on it. This is one example of how mineral salt can affect people.

To wade through the enormity of sulphites, mineral salts, preservatives, and additives, I keep a list of fourteen hundred different foods in my pantry for easy consulting when something new comes into the household.

Sulphites, mineral salts, and preservatives can cause swelling, constipation, diarrhoea, colicky pains, hyperactivity, insomnia, overheating, asthma, sinusitis, hives, itching, rashes, dehydration, bloating, migraines, and feeling excessively thirsty.

## Sulphite Numbers 220-228 and corresponding Names

220 sulphur dioxide
221 sodium sulphite
222 sodium bisulphite
223 sodium metabisulphite
224 potassium metabisulphite
225 potassium sulphite
228 potassium bisulphite

Preservatives such as MSG 621 should be banned due to the severe allergic reactions some people may have, but food manufacturers and some Chinese foods still get away with using it by claiming "no added MSG," but it will still be in the product in other forms.

You will find sulphites mainly in processed, preserved, and fermented products, but you will also find them in shampoo, toothpaste, and fish oil capsules.

## Foods Containing Sulphites

alcoholic beverages
BBQ chicken
baked goods, particularly bread
condiments and relishes
pickled vegetables
olives
white wine vinegar and balsamic vinegar
sugar
frozen meals
modified dairy products
medications
fish and shellfish
gelling agents: gelatin, pectin
jams and jellies
nuts and nut products

desiccated coconut
fruits: dried, glazed, canned, bottled, frozen fruit juices, maraschino cherries
fresh fruits: blueberries, grapes, and plums
processed vegetables: juices, canned, pickled, dried, instant mash, frozen
snack foods: trail mixes, filled crackers
soups: canned, dried
toppings: maple, corn syrup
breakfast cereals, particularly if they contain dried fruits
tea: instant, concentrates
kids ice blocks
packaged fresh meats, cheese, or seafood (best to purchase from the delicatessen)

## Trans Fats

Trans fats are responsible for causing coronary heart disease (the leading cause of death worldwide), high cholesterol, and swelling. On 16 June 2015, the Food and Drug Administration determined that trans fats are not generally recognised as safe and set a three-year time limit for food manufacturers to remove trans fats out of processed foods.

I was astounded to see how many products I had lurking in my cupboard that contained trans fats, and I thought I ate well! All of the products have now been replaced with other brands.

## Foods Containing Trans Fats

Although some bread varieties contain no trans fats, we have found it in different styles by the same manufacturer, so checking the label is necessary.

pita bread
margarine
spreadable butter
breakfast cereals (again, we found it in different styles of cereals by the same manufacturer)

quick-cook noodles
flavoured potato chips
commercial fried chips and foods
frozen battered or crumbed foods
baked goods
pies and pie crusts
commercially packaged nuts
vegetable shortening
cake mixes
frosting
pancake and waffle mixes
ice cream
nondairy creamers
microwave popcorn
mince
cookies
frozen and creamy beverages
meat sticks
crackers
frozen meals
fried Chinese noodles
packaged pudding desserts
tinned and frozen fish
rice purchased in cotton bags
peanut butter
tomato and BBQ sauce
light olive oils
milk
BBQ chicken

Below is where you will find "trans fats" on a nutrition label. It can read

Trans fats < 0.001%, but even this small amount can cause problems over time. I recommend 0 percent.

# Nutrition Facts

**Serving Size 12 grams (2g)**
**Serving Per Container 2**

Amount Per Serving
**Calories  200**

|  | % Daily Values* |
|---|---|
| **Total Fat** 2g | **3%** |
| Saturated Fat 10g | **50%** |
| Trans Fat 8g |  |
| **Sodium** 11mg | **0%** |
| **Total Carbohydrates** 200g | **67%** |
| Dietary Fibre 56g | **224%** |
| Sugars 1g |  |
| **Protein** 39g | **78%** |

*Percent Daily Values are based on a 2,000 calorie diet.

## How I Tackle the "Diet" Debate

I know what you are thinking, because I thought it myself in the beginning. Food and food labelling is so confusing. "What can I eat?" I have patients who ask me sincerely, "Are fruits and vegetables okay to eat?" Everyone seems to be saying something different, and I'm sure it seems that way, but if you look at many diets, like I have, you will find a common denominator: fresh whole foods.

You can't go wrong with fresh fruit and vegetables, combined with plenty of water, whole grains, organic meats, and dairy.

I have studied many diets. Some say vegan is the only way, and that could be true, but I know myself that I like fish, chicken, eggs, and honey, so that diet would not suit me. Diets aren't a "one size fits all." Even though organic food is coming down in cost, it is still expensive for families to eat entirely organic; however, it is something to strive toward.

I read one diet that recommended only eating fruit when it fell off the tree within a thirty-minute time frame, for it to have any nutritional benefits. I was wondering if those people stood under fruit trees all day, just waiting for a snack. I'm sorry, but I don't have time to do that.

This is how I managed to get my head around it all:

I buy the freshest fruit and vegetables as possible from various suppliers. I know the big supermarkets store fruit and vegetables, but it's the freshest and most convenient I can get.

We do grow our own various vegetables, citrus, and herbs; you can't get fresher than that, and I know they haven't been sprayed with pesticides and have been grown organically. We use fresh or dried spices; they are fine to use. We use tinned beans, tomatoes, and sandwich fish for convenience, making sure they contain no sulphites or trans fats.

The only frozen foods we eat are homegrown fruit and vegetables, homemade soups, and homemade meals.

We buy all of our meat fresh, organic or free range.

I drink plenty of filtered fresh water, but if you are not in the habit of drinking water, tap water will do just fine.

You will notice that our recipes have large portion sizes; this is so you can have two nights eating with the one meal. Simply change the carbohydrates and vegetables to make it different, or alternatively, you can freeze the leftover portion for a time when you are rushed and use it as a frozen ready meal.

We never eat take-away foods, and I avoid alcohol, caffeine, sulphites, trans fats, added salt, processed sugars, red meat, and pork products. I also limit my dairy. This was my choice for my digestive system; David and Ben still eat red meat, pork, and dairy.

If I want a sweet treat, we make it at home, and we make it plain with no added icings, jams, syrups, or cream.

We eat limited processed packaged foods, only water crackers and bread; this way, I can check against my list of preservatives and additives to make sure anything new coming into the house is safe, or we take it back.

We found trans fat-free commercial bread, pita bread, cereals, nuts, tinned and frozen fish, rice, oil, peanut butter, and tomato sauce, so we can still enjoy these products.

It's really not that hard. We never threw any food products out; we simply replaced them with the good ones when they were gone.

# Shopping Guide

1. Shop around the outer perimeters of the supermarket. This is where all fresh produce is located; stay away from the middle.
2. Buy fresh fruit and vegetables that are in season; they will be in abundance, cheaper, and at maximum flavour.
3. Buy fresh fruit and vegetables in bulk and freeze it, ready to add to soups and stews or to heat and serve. Cut the kernels off corn and freeze; wipe green beans and freeze (don't blanch first, because this will make them soggy when cooking if using a microwave). Cut tomatoes into eighths and freeze. Squeeze lemons and oranges into ice cube containers. You can pick herbs and freeze in plastic bags. You can also buy in bulk and pickle vegetables, beetroot, cucumber, cabbage, carrots, capsicum/bell peppers, and

onion. (See the recipe for pickling in this book.) Freeze berries for homemade smoothies and sauces.

4. When storing or freezing foods, remember to use BPA-free containers and ziplock bags. BPAs mimic oestrogen, and the body will take it on. This is particularly concerning for hormonal eaters and people who suffer from hormonal conditions. Remember to rinse out your ziplock bags, dry them, and reuse them.

5. Write a shopping list and stick to it. Place the list in a spot that will be in your face, like the refrigerator, and every time you use something out of the pantry or fridge, write it down on the list to restock.

6. Don't shop when you are hungry. My husband and I have our planned morning tea prior to going shopping. This eliminates the need for a coffee and cake while at the shop.

7. Go shopping armed: gather all coupons and write down any specials found in the catalogues prior to shopping. This way, there will be no surprises and added extras; everything will be written on the list beforehand. By going through catalogues and knowing your coupons, you can safely know you are getting your items at the best price, helping you save money. If you don't get catalogues by mail, you can search online.

8. Shop quickly. The more you linger, the more you spend.

9. Shop online. It's quick, it's convenient, and there are no temptations.

10. Only take enough cash to cover your grocery costs.

11. Take a small calculator with you to work out a running tally so you don't go over your budget.

12. Always keep your receipts in a handy spot for approximately a month. You can take back items if they contain preservatives or additives you weren't aware of or if the same product comes on special at another store for less.

13. Ask for a raincheck if the item you want is out of stock.

14. Use your freezer.

15. Nothing should be thrown out or wasted; it can be eaten the next day for lunch, used for the next night's meal, or frozen.

# Holiday Guide

I always seem to have trouble finding quality food that won't upset my stomach while I am on holidays. I picked up the following tips along the way so we can all enjoy our holidays without feeling bloated, uncomfortable, swollen, or thirsty.

## Plane Trips (Regardless of Length)

When booking your ticket, request a vegetarian (or even a vegan) meal. Plane meals are small and designed to make you feel full. They contain a lot of salt due to our tastebuds being off at high altitudes, and it helps to cut costs. Even if you aren't a vegetarian or vegan, it is wise to invest in this practice, just while travelling on the plane. Drink plenty of water while travelling.

## Cruises

I have travelled on a variety of cruise ships and constantly notice people pilling the food onto their plates, only to leave most of it behind. They get up from the table rubbing their stomachs and belching.

The food is buffet style; they need to feed a large number of people on a budget, so they pack it full of mineral salts, preservatives, and additives. You will even find these mineral salts on the table to add extra onto your food. Every item except sweets, cheese, and fresh foods have these salts in them. They also add them to the water they boil food in.

It is illegal to use MSG 621 in food in Australia, which you will find mostly in Asian cooking, but on these cruise ships, they have chefs from various countries who are not aware of the harm they can cause.

The following is a guide to what I eat on a cruise ship:

**Breakfast**

Boiled eggs, toast, fresh tomato and mushrooms, fresh fruit, yoghurt pancakes, bran muffins, cereal, juice, and tea.

**Lunch**

Steamed fish, curry, rice, salads, roasted meat, roasted or steamed vegetables, salads. I usually make up my own salad on a roll, cheese with crackers and nuts, fresh fruit.

**Dinner**

I usually head to the dining room for dinner, because it just seems to be better quality food than the buffet, even though it all comes out of the same galley (even if you go to one of the paying restaurants on board). I usually order seafood, salad, steamed vegetables, or something vegetarian.

## General Holiday Escapes

I generally take my own snack foods with me, even on a short trip.

Most holiday places provide a fridge, so we often take homemade frozen meals along with our microwave to have at night, if we are tired or don't feel like venturing out.

**Breakfast**

We take our own breakfast items, so I know they are safe.

**Lunch**

Head for the local bakery; they will have a fresh selection of ingredients to make up a bread roll of your choice.

Sushi.

Find a supermarket or farmers markets where you can pick up some salad items for a homemade lunch or fresh fruits

Sorbet (treat).

**Dinner**

Clubs are great for a roast meat with vegetables or soup.

Local fish and chip shops generally have grilled fish options or have a burger without the meat and cheese.

Pizza: order a thin vegetarian style with minimal cheese, from a decent establishment, not a food chain.

Tomato-based pastas with seafood or chicken.

Bean burritos with salsa and guacamole.

Chinese vegetable omelettes, soups, long combination soup, chop suey, chow mein, stir-fry, hot pots, and boiled rice.

Lamb *Yeeros* (recipe in this book), with Greek salad and yoghurt.

# Ingredients Used in the Following Recipes

## Proteins

organic mince
nitrate-free eye bacon
stall-free whole pork cuts: loins or boned shoulder
whole organic beef cuts: rump, chuck
whole organic lamb cuts: cutlets, boned leg or shoulder
wild-caught Atlantic salmon or tuna steaks

free-range chicken
free-range eggs
wild-caught hoki
fresh local king prawns
frozen Alaskan king crab
tinned kippers in spring water
tinned tuna in spring water
tinned anchovy fillets

## Dairy

whole milk
natural plain pot set yoghurt
Parmesan cheese
feta cheese
mozzarella cheese
organic butter

## Whole Grains, Pasta, and Beans

wholemeal bread and pita bread
wholemeal pasta
wholemeal flour
wholemeal cous cous
spelt pasta
brown rice or basmati rice
tinned mixed beans
whole oats
bran flakes

## Herbs, Vegetables, Fruits, Nuts, and Seasoning

fresh garden herbs and some dried herbs and spices
Himalayan, sea, or rock salt
cracked black pepper
vegetable-powered stock
vegetables: local, in season and fresh

field mushrooms

curly parsley

carisma white potatoes (low GI)

almonds and walnuts

whole raw coconuts

tinned pineapple, pears, and peaches in natural juice

dried dates

raw sugar

coriander/cilantro

capsicum/bell pepper

**All recipes serve four to six unless stated otherwise
and are trans fat, sulphite, and mineral salt free**

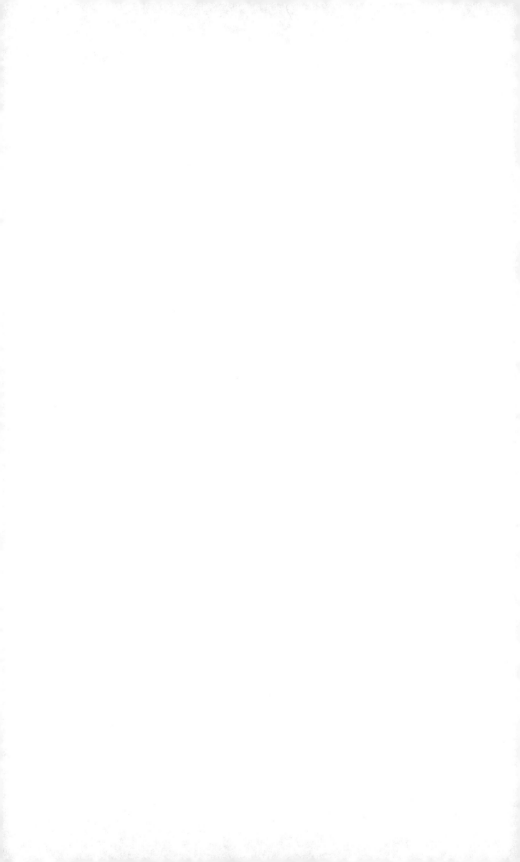

# PART 3

---

# Recipe Index

Anti-inflammatory Plate
Apple Braised Pork Loin with Potato and Onion Pikelets
Aussie Open Sandwich with Char Grilled Potatoes
Baked Fruit Salad
Baked Steak with Tomatoes
Baked Vegetarian Eggplant
Banana Gelato
BBQ Atlantic Salmon on Sweet Potato Boulders with a Garlic-Glazed
Ratatouille Stack
Bean Burritos
Beans 'n' Beans
Beef Gumbo
Beef Stroganoff
Beetroot Salad
BLT Tacos
Breakfast Muesli
Brunch Bread and Butter Pudding
Bubble 'n' Squeak Mash
Capsicum Pear Relish
Cauliflower Cous Cous with Roasted Almonds
Chicken Caesar Patties on Cos Salad
Chicken Pasta Soup
Chicken Skewers with Guilt-Free Satay Dipping Sauce
Chicken Summer Salad
Chicken Tikka Lettuce Cups
Chili Beans
Coconut Crumbed Chicken with Tropical Salad
Cous Cous-Filled Capsicums
Creamy Curried Chicken on Spelt Pasta
Creamy Potato Salad
Crumbed Fish with Sweet and Sour

Curried Chicken
Curried Lamb Stew
Curried Mince Cottage Pie
Curried Prawns with Mini Flatbread
Date and Walnut Cake
Davino's Pasta
Deconstructed Caesar Salad
Easy Sunday Breakfast
Fish in Foil
Fruit Salad Two Ways
Guacca
Herb-Stuffed Chicken with a Mushroom Sauce
Herbed Mini Meat Loaf Sliders with Capsicum Pear Relish
Home-Style Tandoori Chicken
Hot Cos Salad
Hot Prawns on Ribbon Vegetables
Hummus Jingle Bells
Indian-Inspired Potatoes
Indian Stuffed Potatoes with Raita
Italian Pork and Beans
Jaeger Schnitzel with a Pickled Slaw
Khichri
Kristin's Mess
Lamb, Tzatziki, and Tabbouleh Pizza
Lamb Vegetable Soup
Lamb *Yeeros* with Gremolata
Lemon Chicken with Tomatoes
Lemon Potatoes
Lentil Curry
Lo-Carb Cannelloni
Lunchtime Special
Marinated BBQ Vegetables
Meatzza
Mediterranean Medley
Mini Chicken Meatball and Sweet Corn Soup
Moroccan Roasted Vegetables

Nachos with Avocado Salsa
Pickled Slaw
Poached Pears with Almond Walnut Crumble
Prawn Noodle Salad
Prawn Pasta Carbonara
Quick Tomato Soup
Salmon Pasta Salad
Salsa Bonné Bouché
Sautéed Mustard Greens
Savoury Chicken Pie
Seared Tuna Steak on a Vinegar Broccoli Mash
Singapore Noodles
Smoked Nicoise Cups
Southern Herbed Chicken on Bubble 'n' Squeak Mash with
Spaghetti Napolitano with Poached Egg
Spicy Rice Pilaf
Spicy Stuffed Pumpkin
Spring Picnic Slice
Spring Salad
Stir-Fried Vegetables
Stockman's Pepper Stew
Stuffed Steamed Capsicums
Sunset Spritzer
Surf 'n' Turf with Lemon Potatoes and Peas
Tabbouleh and Tzatziki
Thai Crab Appetiser
Thai Tuna Cakes and Salad
Tomato and Onion Bake
Trail Mix
Turmeric Chicken, Cauliflower Cous Cous, and Roasted Almonds
Turmeric Fish with Hot Cos Salad and Potato Boulders
Vegetable Frittata
Vegetable Spaghetti Omelette
Waldorf Salad with Chicken
Zesty Stuffed Mushrooms on Garlic Cabbage

# Anti-Inflammatory Plate

1 Atlantic Salmon Fillet **ai, al, p**
200 g Sweet Potato, peeled and cut into pieces **ai, al, p**
1 Bulb of unpeeled Garlic **ai, al**
3 Broccoli Florets **ai, al**
2 Cauliflower Florets **ai, al, p**
1 Green Tea Bag **ai, al**
Olive Oil **ai, mct**
Parsley to garnish **al, p**
Season to taste **al**

(You can add or swop vegetables with red cabbage, kale and Brussel sprouts.)

Steam, roast, or BBQ Atlantic salmon to liking.

Toss the garlic and sweet potato in a little olive oil.

In a baking dish place the garlic and pieces of sweet potato, cover with foil, and bake at 180º C for 1 hour 15 minutes.

Boil, steam, or microwave broccoli and cauliflower until tender.

Assemble all components onto a plate and garnish with parsley.

Serve with a cup of prepared green tea

Serves 1

# Apple Braised Loin of Pork with Potato and Onion Pikelets

4 x Pork Loins, fat & bone removed, seasoned on both sides **ac, p**
300 ml cloudy Apple Juice **al**
1 Green Apple, peeled and sliced **al**
½ Medium Onion, finely sliced **al**
1 Teaspoon grated Ginger **al, ai**
1 Teaspoon Lemon Zest **al**
2 Teaspoons chopped Sage **al**
1 Teaspoon Hot English Mustard **al**
2½ Tablespoons Butter **neutral**
1 Tablespoon Plain Flour **ac**
Season to taste **al**

In a large pan over med/low heat, add ½ tablespoon butter, add onion and cook until softened, then remove.

Increase heat to med/high and add 2 tablespoons of butter and brown pork for 2 minutes each side; remove from pan.

Stir flour into pan juices to make a paste and slowly add apple juice, ginger, lemon zest, sage, and mustard.

Return onion back to pan and bring to the boil, place in pork and arrange apple over the top of the pork.

Cover and slowly simmer for 10-15 minutes.

<u>Pikelets</u>

600 g Boiled Potatoes, seasoned and mashed with 1 tablespoon of butter and enough milk to make a firm consistency **ac, p**

Add ½ Medium Onion, finely chopped **al**

When mash and onion mix is cold, form 8 pikelets.

Cook in a lightly oiled pan over medium heat until browned on both sides.

# Aussie Open Sandwich with Char-Grilled Potatoes

2 Slices Bread **ac**
1 Beef Mince Pattie, seasoned **ac, p**
1 Egg **al**
¼ Onion, sliced **al**
1 Slice Pineapple **al, p**
¼ Cup shredded Lettuce **al**
1 Tablespoon grated Carrot **al**
2 Slices Tomato **al, p**
2 Slices Beetroot **ac**
6 Potatoes, peeled, quartered, and partially cooked until tender **al, p**
1 Tablespoon Olive Oil **mct, ai**
Season to taste **al**

Cook mince, egg, onion, and pineapple on a BBQ plate.

Coat potatoes in seasoned olive oil and place on the char grill to heat through and get a slight char colouring.

Toast bread.

Assemble the cold components on one piece of toast and the hot components on the other piece of toast.

Serve with the char-grilled potatoes.

***"These are my healthy chips!"***

# Baked Fruit Salad

1 x 425 g tin each of Pineapple, Pears, and Peaches in Natural Juice, strained and diced **al, p**

Topping

¾ Cup Plain Flour **ac**
2 Tablespoons Butter **neutral**
½ Cup blitzed Fresh Coconut **al**
¼ Cup Sugar **ac**

Sift the flour into a bowl, rub in the butter, and combine with the coconut and sugar.

Place the fruit medley in a 1.5 litre baking dish and cover with the topping.

Bake at 180º C for 30 minutes or until the top is browned.

Serve with finely sliced mint **al.**

# Baked Steak with Tomatoes

750 g Rump Steak **ac, p**
1 Medium Onion, sliced **al**
2 Cloves Garlic, chopped **ai, al**
1 Small Chili, chopped **al**
2 Tablespoons chopped Parsley **al, p**
1 Teaspoon chopped Rosemary **al**
4 Large Tomatoes, cut into eighths **al, p**
½ Teaspoon Stock, dissolved in a little water **al**
3 Tablespoons Plain Flour **ac,** seasoned **al**
Season to taste **al**

Remove the fat from the steak and cut into large pieces.

Flour steak and place in a casserole dish with a lid.

Sprinkle onions, garlic, chili, parsley, and rosemary over the steak.

Place in tomatoes and pour over stock. Season again.

Place into a pre-heated 180º C oven for 1½ hours.

Serve with crusty bread, rice, or cous cous.

# Baked Vegetarian Eggplant

2 Eggplants, split lengthways, remove half the flesh from each half and reserve **al**
4 Medium Mushrooms, sliced and diced **al**
¼ Red Capsicum, finely diced **al**
1 Cup of tightly packed shredded Spinach **al, p**
1 Tomato, diced **al, p**
⅓ Cup Feta Cheese **ac**
½ Small Onion, finely diced **al**
1 Clove Garlic, crushed **ai, al**
1 Tablespoon Olive Oil **mct, ai**
900 g Peeled Sweet Potato, boiled and mashed **ai, al, p**
Season to taste **al**

Sprinkle eggplant hulls and removed flesh with salt and leave for 30 minutes.

Wash the salt off and pat dry. Dice the removed flesh.

In a pan over med/low heat, add oil, onion, and garlic, cook for 3 minutes, then add diced eggplant, capsicum, and mushrooms and cook for a further 3 minutes.

Add spinach and seasoning and cook for a further 5 minutes.

Cool mixture.

Mix in tomato and feta cheese.

Divide mixture between the eggplant hulls and place into an oven-proof dish.

Cover with foil and bake at 200° C for 60-75 minutes.

Serve on a bed of sweet potato mash.

# Banana Gelato

3 Ripe Bananas **al, p**
2 Tablespoons Honey **al**
2 Tablespoons Lemon Juice **al**
1 Teaspoon Cinnamon **al**
2 Passion fruits, pulped **al**

Cut bananas up into chunks, place in a plastic bag, and freeze until solid.

In a food processor add the bananas, honey, cinnamon, and lemon juice and blend until smooth.

Spoon into four individual ramekin dishes and return to the freezer until frozen.

For best results, leave overnight.

Top with passion fruit pulp.

*"I eat this for a dessert or during the day for a healthy snack."*

# BBQ Atlantic Salmon on Sweet Potato Boulders with a Garlic-Glazed Ratatouille Stack

1 Atlantic Salmon Fillet **mct, ai, p**
2 Thick slices Tomato **al, p**
1 Thick slice Onion **al**
1 Thick slice Zucchini **ac, p**
1 Extra Thick Slice Sweet Potato, cut into 4 **al, ai, p**
1 Clove Garlic, crushed **ai, al**
2 Tablespoons Olive Oil **mct, ai**
Season to taste **al**

Combine olive oil and garlic and set aside to infuse for 2 hours.

Steam, boil, or microwave sweet potato until tender.

Pre-heat the BBQ for 5 minutes.

Place the fish on the BBQ plate along with the tomato, zucchini, and onion.

Flip the tomato, onion, and zucchini over when tender and brush with olive oil and garlic mixture and cook for a further 1-2 minutes.

Cook fish for 4-6 minutes each side, depending on thickness and preference.

Place the sweet potato on the char grill until heated through and slightly charred.

Serves 1.

# Bean Burritos

2 x 420 g Tin Bean Mix **ac, p**
1 Medium Onion, 3 Cloves Garlic, and 1 Stick Celery,
finely chopped **al, ai**
1 x 400 g Tin Tomatoes, crushed + juice **al, p**
2 Tablespoons Tomato Paste **al, p**
1 Teaspoon Stock Powder **ac**
3 Chilies, chopped **al**
2 Teaspoons Paprika **al**
1 Teaspoon Sugar **ac**
1 Tablespoon Olive Oil **mct, ai**
1 x Packet 5-7 Pita Breads **ac**

Season to taste **al**

Rinse bean mix and set aside.

Add olive oil to the pan; add onion, celery, garlic, and seasoning; cook until vegetables are soft.

Add tomatoes + juice, tomato paste, stock, chilies, sugar, and paprika. Bring to the simmer, adjust seasoning, add beans, mix through, cover, and cook for 1½ hours.

Remove lid and simmer to reduce and thicken.

Cool mixture.

Spoon cooled bean mixture onto pita breads, careful not to overfill, roll up, and place onto an oven tray, folded side down.

Bake on 160º C for approximately 20-30 minutes or until golden, crunchy, and heated through.

Serve with garden salad or finely sliced lettuce **al,** salsa **al,** guacca **al, p,** yoghurt neutral **p,** and baked pita chips (recipe under Nachos with Avocado Salsa; Guacca and Salsa recipe in this book).

# Beans 'n' Beans

250 g Green Beans **al**
2 Teaspoons Lemon Juice **al**
½ Tin 5 Bean Mix **ac, p**
½ Teaspoon Mustard Powder **al**
1 Tablespoon finely chopped Onion **al**
1 Teaspoon Sugar **ac**
1 Tablespoon finely chopped Parsley **al, p**
1 Teaspoon Olive Oil **mct, ai**
2 Tablespoons White Vinegar **ac**
Season to taste **al**

Slice beans and add to a salted pot of boiling water, cook for 2-3 minutes or until just tender, remove, and plunge into cold water.

Set aside to dry in a colander.

Wash the brine from the bean mix in colander and set aside to dry.

Blend vinegar, lemon juice, mustard, sugar, olive oil, and seasoning together in a small bowl.

Combine all ingredients, including onion and parsley, and cover.

Refrigerate for 2 hours.

*"**This is a wonderful accompaniment to go with cooked meats or a simple vegetarian lunch option.**"*

# Beef Gumbo

500-750 g Chuck Steak **ac, p**
1 Large Onion, sliced **al**
2 x 400 g Tinned Tomatoes + Juice **al, p**
4 Teaspoons Curry Powder **al**
2 Teaspoons Sugar **ac**
3 Tablespoons Plain Flour, seasoned **ac**
4 Tablespoons Olive Oil **mct, ai**
Season to taste **al**

Remove fat from the steak and cut into 3 cm cubes. Dust steak with seasoned flour.

Heat large pot over medium heat, add 1 tablespoon of oil and the sliced onion, cook until slightly soft, remove from pot, and set aside.

Add remaining oil and steak, brown all over and reduce heat to medium, add the curry powder, and stir to coat the steak.

Return the cooked onion to the pot and mix through.

Add tomatoes, juice, and sugar, bring up to a slow simmer, and adjust the seasoning.

Cover and cook for 2½-3 hours.

Serve with a dollop of natural yoghurt **neutral, p**, in a bowl or on top of rice or cous cous with some greens.

# Beef Stroganoff

500-750 g Chuck Steak **ac, p**
2 Onions, sliced **ai, al**
2 Tablespoons Tomato Paste **al, p**
1 Cup Stock **ac**
3 Tablespoons chopped Parsley **al, p**
3 Tablespoons Plain Flour **ac,** seasoned **al**
4 Tablespoons Olive Oil **mct, ai**
4-6 Mushrooms, quartered **al**
Season to taste **al**

Remove any fat from steak and cut into 3 cm cubes.

Cook onions until slightly soft and remove from the pan.

Dust the steak with seasoned flour.

Add olive oil to the pan and brown the meat on medium heat.

Return the cooked onions to the pan and add tomato paste, stirring to combine.

Pour in the stock, adding parsley and seasoning.

Slowly simmer for 2½-3 hours, adding the mushrooms in the final

15 minutes before serving.

Serve with natural yoghurt **neutral, p**, in a bowl or on top of rice or crusty bread with some greens.

*"I like to eat this without the meat portion so David adds extra mushrooms for me. He dishes up the meat first for him and Ben and then I get the mushrooms with sauce."*

# Beetroot Salad

Bunch Baby Beetroots, trimmed **al**
¼ Cup crushed Walnuts **mct, ai**
½ Cup Feta Cheese, crumbled **ac**
Pinch of Sugar **ac**

<u>Vinaigrette</u>

2 Tablespoons White Vinegar **ac**
1 Teaspoon Lemon Juice **al**
1 Teaspoon Sugar **ac**
1 Teaspoon Olive Oil **mct, ai**
Season to taste **al**

Combine in a bowl and set aside

Wrap beetroots in foil, roast on 180° C, for approximately 1 hour or until tender, inserting a skewer into the middle to check.

Cool slightly and peel.

Set aside until completely cooled down.

Slice into wedges and toss in bowl with the vinaigrette and another small pinch of sugar.

Top with walnuts and feta and a drizzle of olive oil.

> *"This is a great accompaniment to cooked meats or, by adding a leafy green such as spinach or kale, may be used as an all-round lunch salad, sneaking in extra vegetables."*

# BLT Tacos

4 Eyes of Bacon, chopped **ac, p**
1 Tablespoon Olive Oil **mct, ai**
4 Iceberg Lettuce Leaves, sliced into ribbons **al**
1 Avocado, sliced **mct, ai, al, p**
2 Tomatoes, split and sliced **al**
4 Tortillas **ac**

Fry bacon in olive oil until browned and drain on paper towel.

Spread the entire tortilla with mustard spread, place in lettuce, and top with tomato, avocado, and bacon.

Mustard Spread

2 Tablespoons Yoghurt **neutral, p**
2 Teaspoons Hot English Mustard **al**

Blend all ingredients together well.

***"This is a great dish for lunch."***

# Breakfast Muesli

3 Cups Rolled Oats **ac, p**
2 Cups, slightly crushed Bran **ac, p**
⅓ Cup Shredded Coconut **al**
2 Tablespoons Sesame Seeds **ac**
⅓ Cup crushed Almonds **mct, al, p**
1 Tablespoon Butter **neutral**
2 Tablespoons Olive Oil **mct, ai**
3 Tablespoons Honey **al**
¼ Cup chopped Dates **al, p**
⅓ Cup Sultanas **al, p**

Pre-heat oven to 170° C.

Blend all dry ingredients together except the dates and sultanas.

Melt the honey, oil, and butter in a saucepan and mix through the dry ingredients.

Place the mixture onto a baking tray and bake for 35-40 minutes, stirring every 5-10 minutes.

Cool.

Add the dates and sultanas and seal in an airtight container.

Serve with fresh fruit **al** and sweetened natural yoghurt **neutral, p.**

# Brunch Bread and Butter Pudding

3-4 Medium Potatoes **ac, p**
1 Bunch Asparagus **al**
1 Leek, sliced **al**
2 Eyes of Bacon, sliced **ac, p**
1 Tablespoon Butter **neutral**
6 Eggs **al**
3 Cups Milk **ac, p**
3-4 Slices Bread **ac**
Season with Salt and Cracked Black Pepper **al**

Garlic Butter:

1 Tablespoon Butter **neutral**
1 Small Clove Garlic, crushed **ai, al**

Combine ingredients together.

Peel and cut potatoes in halves and steam, boil, or microwave until tender.

Blanch asparagus in salted water for 2-3 minutes, remove and plunge into cold water, and cut into 1 cm pieces.

Cook the leek in butter over medium/low heat until softened.

Slice potatoes into thick slices and place into a 2 litre baking dish, season with cracked black pepper.

Spread over the leeks then the asparagus.

Spread the bread with the garlic butter.

Beat together the eggs and milk and season well.

Pour the egg and milk mixture over the bread and set aside for 30 minutes; this allows the bread to soak up some of the liquid.

Place the bread on a pan, buttered side facing upward, and scatter bacon over top.

Bake at 180º C for 40-50 minutes.

Bread should be golden and puffed up in the middle.

Serves 6

# Bubble 'n' Squeak Mash

700 g peeled Sweet Potato **ai, al, p**
300 g Pumpkin **al, p**
300 g Carrots **al**
1 Clove Garlic **ai, al**
½ Cup Peas **al**
½ Cup Corn **al**
Season to taste **al**

Boil sweet potato, pumpkin, carrots, and garlic until soft; mash together and season.

Boil peas and corn separately until cooked and mix through mash.

This accompanies the Southern Herbed Chicken (recipe in this book) or can be eaten as a separate vegetarian dish.

**"This recipe can also be used as a baby food."**

# Capsicum Pear Relish

100 ml Brown Vinegar **ac**
3 Tablespoons Sugar **ac**
½ Teaspoon Yellow Mustard Seeds **al**
½ Green Apple, finely diced **al**
½ Pear, finely diced **al**
½ Red and Green Capsicum, finely diced **al**

Heat vinegar, sugar, and mustard seeds in a medium pot for 5 minutes, or until the sugar dissolves and mixture boils.

Add remaining ingredients.

Bring to the boil.

Reduce heat and simmer, uncovered, for 30 minutes.

Serve cold as a pickle relish on hamburgers or with Herbed Mini Meatloaf Sliders (recipe in this book).

## Cauliflower Cous Cous with Roasted Almonds

2 Cups blitzed raw Cauliflower **al, ai**
2 Tablespoons Butter **neutral**
2 Dozen Almonds **mct, al, p**
Season to taste **al**

In a pan on medium heat add the butter and cook the cauliflower with seasoning for 1 minute.

Crush and roast the almonds on a baking tray at 180° for 3-5 minutes.

Sprinkle almonds over the top of the cous cous to garnish.

*"This is a wonderful side dish and alternative to rice or pasta."*

# Chicken Caesar Patties on Cos Salad

500 g Chicken Mince **al, p**
½ Cup Bread Crumbs **ac**
4 Eyes Bacon, finely diced **ac, p**
2 Tablespoons Dijon Mustard **ac**
1 Clove Garlic, crushed **ai, al**
Season to taste **al**
1 Baby Cos Lettuce **al**
4 Anchovy Fillets **ac**
4 Eggs, hard boiled and mashed **al**

Parmesan Cheese (small amount), shaved **ac**

Combine mince, bread crumbs, bacon, mustard, garlic, and seasoning.

Roll into 12 patties and cook.

Arrange lettuce on a plate, place on patties, scatter around egg, and sprinkle with cheese.

Top with an anchovy fillet.

# Chicken Pasta Soup

3 Full Chicken Frames **al, p**
1,750 ml Water
1 Large Onion and 2 sticks Celery, diced **ai, p, al**
2 Carrots and 1 Parsnip, grated **al, p**
1 Tablespoon chopped Parsley **al, p**
50 g Linguine Pasta **ac**
Season to taste **al**


In a large boiler place in chicken frames and water; bring to the boil, skim the surface of any scum, reduce heat, and simmer covered for

1 hour.

Remove chicken frames and set aside to cool, slightly.

Strain the broth and return to pot along with the rest of the ingredients, simmer, covered for 1 hour.

Meanwhile, remove flesh from chicken frames and refrigerate.

Return the chicken meat to broth at the end of the cooking time, heat through, and season.

**"*This is your ideal Chicken Broth with Vegetables, great for healing.*"**

# Chicken Skewers with Guilt-Free Satay Dipping Sauce

800 g Skinless Chicken Thigh Fillets **al, p**
8 Pineapple Rings **al, p**

<u>Satay Sauce</u>

3 Tablespoons Yoghurt **neutral, p**
1 Tablespoon Tahini Paste **ac**
½ Tablespoon Curry Powder **ac**
¾ Tablespoon Sugar **ac**
1 Tablespoon Pineapple Juice **al**
Pinch Salt **al**

Mix all sauce ingredients together.

Place chicken on pre-soaked bamboo skewers.

Cook chicken on char grill along with pineapple rings.

*"This is a good entertaining recipe and can accompany
the Marinated Vegetables for a complete dinner."*

# Chicken Summer Salad

2 Cups cooked, shredded Chicken **al, p**
2 Oranges, segmented **al**
½ Red Capsicum, sliced **al**
1 Stick Celery, sliced **al, ai**
½ Cup, finely sliced Fennel **al, ai, p**
2 Cups, shredded Lettuce **al**

Combine chicken, orange, capsicum, celery, fennel, and lettuce in a bowl.

Pour over dressing and toss just before serving.

<u>Dressing</u>

¼ Cup Orange Juice **al**
1 Tablespoon Lemon Juice **al**
1 Teaspoon, grated Lemon Rind **al**
2 Teaspoons Honey **al**
1 Tablespoon Olive Oil **mct, ai**
2 Tablespoons chopped Parsley **al, p**
2 Shallots, sliced **al**

Pinch of Salt **al**

Blend all ingredients together and set aside.

*"I love this salad; it is so fresh and healthy."*

# Chicken Tikka Lettuce Cups

300 g Skinless Chicken Thigh Fillets, diced into 2 cm pieces **al, p**
2 Cloves Garlic, 1 chopped **ai, al**
1 Iceberg Lettuce, separated into cups **al**
3 Tablespoons Olive Oil **mct, ai**
1 Chili, roughly chopped **al**
400 g Tin Tomatoes **al**
1 Teaspoon grated Ginger **ai, al**
½ Medium Onion, diced **al**
½ Teaspoon Paprika **al**
1 Red Capsicum, diced **al**
1 Teaspoon Ground Coriander **al**
½ Teaspoon Turmeric **ai, al**

Pinch Cumin **al**

½ Teaspoon Sugar **ac**
2 Tablespoons chopped Coriander **al**
Season to taste **al**

In a mortar and pestle, grind together 1 clove garlic, chili, 1 tablespoon oil, pinch of salt and pepper, ginger, paprika, ground coriander, and cumin to make a paste. Transfer to a bowl, add the chicken, and coat well. Cover and marinate for a minimum of 2 hours.

In a pan over medium heat, add 1 tablespoon oil, onion, capsicum, 1 clove garlic, and turmeric; cook until softened. Add coriander, cooking for a further 1 minute; add tomatoes, sugar, and season.

Cover and slowly simmer.

In another pan over high heat, add 1 tablespoon of oil and stir-fry the chicken for 2-3 minutes, then add directly to the sauce. Cover and slowly simmer for 30 minutes. Remove lid, increase heat, and simmer for a further 30 minutes until sauce is thick.

Place a small amount of mixture into lettuce cups and top with yoghurt **neutral, p.**

*"This is a meal that needs only hands to eat!"*

# Chili Beans

500 g Beef Mince **ac, p**
1 Medium Onion, 3 Cloves Garlic and 1 Stick Celery,
finely chopped **al, ai**
1 x 400 g Tin Tomatoes, crushed + juice **al, p**
2 Tablespoons Tomato Paste **al, p**
1 Teaspoon Stock Powder **ac**
3 Chilies, chopped **al**
2 Teaspoons Paprika **al**
1 Teaspoon Sugar **ac**
1 x 420 g Tin Bean Mix **ac, p**
Season to taste **al**

Rinse bean mix and set aside. Brown mince in pan over high heat, reduce to med/low heat, and drain excess liquid.

Push mince to one side of pan, add onion, celery, garlic, and seasoning, cook until vegetables are soft.

Combine vegetables and mince, add tomatoes + juice, tomato paste, stock, chilies, sugar, and paprika. Bring to the simmer, adjust seasoning, add beans, mix through, cover, and cook for 1½ hours.

Remove lid and simmer for a further 30 minutes to thicken.

Serve with finely sliced lettuce **al**, salsa **al**, guacca **al, p,** yoghurt **neutral, p,** and baked pita chips (recipe under Nachos with Avocado Salsa). (Guacca and Salsa recipe in this book).

NB: I leave out the mince in this recipe to make it a vegetarian dish.

Add two tins of beans, instead of 1 tin, and leave out the cooking method for the mince. Sweat the vegetables off in a little olive oil, firstly, and then add the tomatoes with the rest of the ingredients, and lastly the beans go in.

*"We sometimes break up a whole cos lettuce and*
*spoon the bean mixture into the cups and top with*
*salsa and yoghurt; we call this Taco Boats."*

# Coconut Crumbed Chicken with Tropical Salad

500 g Chicken Tenderloins **al, p**
½ Cup Blitzed Coconut **al**
½ Cup Breadcrumbs **ac**
¼ Cup Plain Flour, seasoned **ac**
1 Egg **al**
½ Cup Milk **ac, p**
Olive Oil for frying **mct, ai**
4 Small Mangoes **al**
1 Tin Pineapple Rings **al, p**
¼ Cup finely sliced Mint leaves **al**
¼ Cup Lemon Juice **al**
1 Chili to taste **al**

Combine coconut and breadcrumbs. Beat together egg and milk. Lightly flour chicken and dip into egg wash, place into crumbs and coat both sides, pressing firmly. Fry until golden on both sides.

Salad

Remove cheeks from mangoes, scoop out flesh with a spoon, and slice lengthways. Halve pineapple rings and slice finely. Finely slice chili and mint leaves.

Assemble by layering mango and pineapple and top with chili and mint.

*"A meal for someone who has a sweet tooth."*

# Cous Cous-Filled Capsicums

2 Red Capsicums **al**
1 Cup Cous Cous **ac**
(Cooked to packet directions with stock and cooled)
1 Teaspoon Butter **neutral**
1 Egg, boiled, cooled, and mashed **al**
½ Small Onion, finely diced **al**
Chili to taste, finely diced **al**
2 Medium Mushrooms, diced **al**
1 Cup tightly packed, shredded Spinach **al, p**
1 Teaspoon chopped Thyme **al**
2 Tablespoons Olive Oil **mct, ai**
Season to taste **al**

Split capsicums lengthways and remove membrane.

Cook onion in 1 tablespoon of oil until soft.

Add another 1 tablespoon of oil, mushrooms, thyme, and spinach.

Season and cook for a further 5-6 minutes.

Set aside to cool.

Combine cooled mixture with cous cous and egg.

Spoon and press lightly into capsicums.

Place in an oven-proof dish, cover with foil, and cook at 200° C for 1 hour.

**NB**

When cooking the cous cous, add 1 teaspoon of butter before adding stock. When absorption has taken place, fork through to fluff.

*"This is one of my favourite vegetarian dishes."*

# Creamy Curried Chicken on Spelt Pasta

400 g Spelt Pasta **ac**
300 g (leftover), Chicken, shredded **al, p**
1 Small Onion, diced **ac**
½ Stick Celery, diced **al, p, ai**
1 Clove Garlic, finely chopped **ai, al**
1 Tablespoon chopped Parsley **al, p**
1 Teaspoon Curry Powder **al**
1 Tablespoon Plain Flour **ac**
1 Teaspoon Sugar **ac**
½ Tablespoon Butter **neutral**
¾ Cup Milk **ac, p**
¾ Cup Stock **ac**
1 Teaspoon Lemon Juice **al**
Season to taste **al**

Heat pan over med/low heat, add the butter, onion, celery, garlic, and seasoning.

Cook until vegetables are slightly soft.

Add the flour and curry, stir to coat all vegetables, cook for 1 minute.

Blend the milk and stock together and start to add a little at a time, while stirring, to avoid lumps.

Add sugar, lemon juice, parsley, and chicken.

Bring to a slow simmer and adjust seasoning.

Cover and cook for 30-40 minutes.

Stir occasionally and add more milk if mixture becomes too thick.

Serve with extra Lemon **al.**

***"This recipe came from my Nan; it was one of her favourite recipes."***

# Creamy Potato Salad

800 g Peeled Potatoes **ac, p**
3 Eyes Bacon, diced **ac, p**
¼ Medium Onion, finely diced **al**
½ Avocado **mct, ai, al, p**
2 Tablespoons Yoghurt **neutral, p**
2 Teaspoons Lemon Juice **al**
2 Boiled Eggs, chopped **al**
1 Teaspoon Olive Oil **mct, ai**
Salt **al**
Shallots, finely sliced **al**

Cut potatoes into 1.5-2 cm cubes, boil in salted water until tender, drain, and rinse under cold water.

Refrigerate until cold.

Slightly brown bacon in olive oil. Remove, drain on paper towel, and cool.

Roughly mash avocado, add lemon juice and salt, and mash until smooth. Blend through yoghurt.

In a bowl, mix together the avocado mixture, onion, and bacon.

Add potato and fold through until coated, then gently fold in egg.

Garnish with shallots. **al**

*"I have this with a piece of grilled Atlantic salmon."*

# Crumbed Fish with Sweet and Sour

8 Hoki Fillets **ac, p,** crumbed and pan fried in olive oil **mct, ai**
1 Medium Onion, sliced **al**
2 Tablespoons Tomato Paste **al, p**
¼ Red Capsicum, chopped **al**
2 Teaspoons Stock Powder **ac**
1 Stick Celery, chopped **al, ai, p**
1 Tablespoon Sugar **ac**
1 Medium Carrot, split and sliced **al**
1 Cup Water
4 Pineapple Rings, chopped + Juice **al**
½ Tablespoon White Vinegar **ac**
1 Tablespoon Corn Flour **ac**
1 Tablespoon Olive Oil **mct, ai**
Season to taste **al**

In a pan, over med/low heat, add oil and place in onion, capsicum, celery, carrot, and seasoning, and cook until vegetables soften slightly.

Add water, pineapple juice, stock, tomato paste, sugar, and vinegar; bring to a simmer; and add pineapple.

In a small bowl, blend corn flour in a little water; stir into vegetables to thicken slightly. Adjust seasoning.

Cook uncovered for 15-20 minutes or until vegetables are just tender.

*"You can also use the sweet and sour sauce with any meats or just on its own over rice."*

# Curried Chicken

3-4 Chicken Thighs **al, p**
3 Teaspoons Curry Powder **al**
1 Large Onion, diced **al**
3 Tablespoons Plain Flour **ac**
1 Stick Celery, diced **al, ai, p**
500 ml Stock **al**
¼ Red Capsicum, diced **al**
1 Tablespoon Olive Oil **mct, ai**
1 Carrot, split and sliced **al**
3 Tablespoons chopped Parsley **al, p**
½ Green Apple, diced **al**
¼ Cup Peas **al**
Season to taste **al**

Cook vegetables and apple in a pot over medium heat, until soft.

Add curry powder and flour, mix to coat all ingredients, and cook for 1 minute.

Add stock slowly while stirring to thicken; add parsley and seasoning.

Bring to the boil and place in the chicken, reduce to a slow simmer, cover, and cook for 1½ hours.

Remove chicken and shred, return to pot with peas for a further 30 minutes.

*"A regular weekly staple for us."*

# Curried Lamb Stew

500 g Lamb, chopped into chunks & tossed in 3 tablespoons seasoned plain flour **ac**
1 Teaspoon each of Turmeric **al, ai** and Paprika **al**
½ Teaspoon Cumin **al**
2 Teaspoons each of Ground Coriander **al** and Sugar **ac**
1 Large Onion, chopped **al**
2 x 400 g tins Tomatoes + Juice, crushed **al, p**
2 Cloves Garlic, crushed **ai, al**
3 Tablespoons chopped Parsley **al, p**
2 Carrots and 1 Stick Celery, diced **ai, p, al**
4 Tablespoons Olive Oil **mct, ai**
Chili to taste **al**
Season to taste **al**

In a large pot over med/low heat, add 1 tablespoon of oil and cook onion, garlic, celery, carrot, and chili until tender; remove from pan and set aside.

Increase heat to medium, add 3 tablespoons of oil, and brown the Lamb.

Scatter turmeric, cumin, coriander, and paprika over top and stir to coat.

Return vegetables along with tomatoes, sugar, and parsley.

Season and slowly simmer, covered, for 2 hours.

Serve with yoghurt **neutral, p** and rice or cous cous and greens.

# Curried Mince Cottage Pie

500 g Beef Mince **ac, p**
3 Tablespoons chopped Parsley **al, p**
1 Medium Onion, diced **al**
3 Teaspoons Curry Powder **al**
½ Green Apple, diced **al**
2 Tablespoons Plain Flour **ac**
1 Stick Celery, diced **al, p, ai**
1½ Cups Stock **al**
¼ Red Capsicum, diced **al**
1 Carrot, diced **al**
Season to taste **al**

## Topping

6 Medium Potatoes (mashed with milk) **ac, p**

Brown mince over high heat, move to one side, and drain off fat.

Add apple and vegetables to opposite side of pan and cook on med/low heat until tender.

Combine vegetables and mince, add curry powder and flour, stir to coat all ingredients, and cook for a further 1 minute.

Add stock, slowly while stirring, to thicken. Add parsley and season.

Simmer, covered, on low for 1½ hours, stirring occasionally to prevent sticking.

Spoon mince into ramekins.

Cover mince with potato mash and place under grill until golden.

# Curried Prawns with Mini Flatbread

500 g Cooked Prawns **ac**
600 ml Water
1 Medium Onion, diced **al**
1 Stick Celery, diced **al, p, ai**
¼ Red Capsicum, diced **al**
1 Carrot, split and sliced **al**
½ Green Apple, diced **al**
2 Teaspoons Curry Powder **al**
2 Tablespoons Plain Flour **ac**
3 Tablespoons chopped Parsley **al, p**
1 Tablespoon Olive Oil **mct, ai**
Season to taste **al**

Peel prawns and place heads in a pot with the 600 ml of water, simmer for 1 hour, then crush with a potato masher and strain.

You will be left with approximately 400 ml of stock.

Over med/low heat, place oil in a pan with vegetables, apple, and parsley, cook until tender.

Stir in curry powder and flour to coat all vegetables and slowly add the stock, while stirring to thicken. Bring to a simmer, add prawns, cover, and cook for 50-60 minutes.

Mini Flatbreads

¼ Cup Yoghurt **neutral, p** to ½ Cup Self-Raising Flour **ac**

Combine with a knife; knead for 30 seconds.

Cut into 8 equal pieces and roll out on a floured surface to ½ mm. thickness.

Cook on high heat for 2 minutes, turn over and heat for a further minute.

*"The mini flatbreads can be made bigger for pizza bases, used for tacos or as pita chips, or to replace traditional bread, rice, or cous cous."*

# Date and Walnut Cake

1 Cup chopped Dates **al, p**
¾ Cup Boiling Water
1 Teaspoon Bi-Carbonate Soda **al**
60 g Butter **neutral**
1 Cup Sugar **ac**
1 Egg **al**
¼ Teaspoon Vanilla Essence **ac**
1 Cup Plain Flour, sifted **ac**
½ Cup Self-Raising Flour, sifted **ac**
½ Cup chopped Walnuts **mct, ai, ac**

Combine dates, boiling water, and bi-carbonate soda and stand until cold.

Cream together butter and sugar and then mix in egg and vanilla essence.

Stir in date mixture, fold in combined, sifted flours, and add walnuts.

Grease and line a loaf tin, pour in ingredients and cook in a moderate oven 180° C for 60-70 minutes.

After 30 minutes, cover with foil, to protect top from burning.

Serve with herbal tea. **al**

# Davino's Pasta

375 g Dry Spaghetti **ac**
3 Rashes Bacon, sliced **ac, p**
1 Small Onion, diced **al**
3 Large Cloves Garlic, crushed **ai, al**
3-4 Medium Mushrooms, quartered **al**
½ Tomato, diced **al, p**
Scattering of Peas **al**
1 Teaspoon each of chopped Thyme and Basil **al**
1 Tablespoon chopped Parsley **al, p**
8 Tablespoons Olive Oil **mct, ai**
Chili to taste **al**
Season with Salt and Cracked Black Pepper **al**

Over med/low heat, add oil, onion, garlic, bacon, chili, thyme, basil, parsley, and season.

Cook for 10 minutes or until tender.

Add mushrooms and cook for a further 5 minutes.

Add peas and cook for another 5 minutes.

Toss through tomato and serve with a sprinkle of

Parmesan cheese **ac**

# Deconstructed Caesar Salad

2 Slices Bread **ac**
½ Clove Garlic **ai, al**
1 Teaspoon Dijon Mustard **ac**
2 Eyes Bacon **ac, p**
2 Large Cos Lettuce leaves **al**
1 Egg, boiled and quartered **al**
2 Anchovy Fillets **ac**
Parmesan Cheese, shaved **ac**

Cook bacon.

Toast bread and rub with garlic, smear with mustard.

Place on bacon, lettuce cup, Parmesan, and the two egg quarters on each piece.

Top with an anchovy fillet.

Serves 2

# Easy Sunday Breakfast

4 Large Field Mushrooms **al**
4 Eggs **al**
1 Tablespoon chopped Parsley **al, p**
2 Eyes of Bacon, finely diced **ac, p**
¼ Medium Onion, finely diced **al**
½ Tomato, finely diced **al, p**
Season with Salt and Cracked Black Pepper **al**

On a lined and oiled oven tray, place peeled mushrooms.

Crack an egg into each mushroom cup.

Divide over parsley, bacon, onion, and tomato; top with cracked black pepper; and season to taste.

Bake at 180° C for 20-30 minutes, depending on egg preference.

***"I leave the bacon off to make it vegetarian."***

# Fish in Foil

1 Fillet of White Fish **al, p**
¼ Cup cooked Rice **ac,**
¼ Cup grated Zucchini **al, p**
2 Tablespoons grated Carrot **al**
3 Thin slices of Onion **al**
1 Thick slice of Tomato **al, p**
½ Teaspoon Butter **neutral**
¼ Teaspoon Dried Tarragon **al**
1 Teaspoon chopped Parsley **al, p**
Season with Salt and Cracked Black Pepper **al**
1 Thin Lemon Slice **al**

In the centre of a large sheet of foil, place the rice and spread out to a circle 1 cm thick.

Top with zucchini, carrot, onion, tomato, and then fish.

Smear the butter on top of the fish; sprinkle with tarragon, parsley, and seasoning; and top with lemon slice.

Wrap up in a parcel and bake at 180° C for 20 minutes.

Serves 1

# Fruit Salad Two Ways

## Fruit Used

½ Punnet Strawberries, washed, green removed, and halved **al**
2 Kiwi Fruit, peeled and sliced into eighths **al**
1 Ripe Banana, sliced on the diagonal **al, p**
Any Fruits may be used.

## Crepes

1 Cup Plain Flour **ac**
1¼ Cups Milk **ac, p**
1 Egg **al**
30 g Butter, melted **neutral**

Sift flour into a bowl; make a well in the middle. Whisk together the milk, egg, and butter; pour into the well; and mix together to make a smooth batter.

Rest for 30 minutes.

Pre-heat a pan or skillet on high and lightly grease before each pancake with butter.

Using a ¼ measuring cup, fill with batter and place into pan, swirling the batter around to form a thin, covered layer.

When the edges start to curl, flip over and cook for a further 1-2 minutes. Repeat for each pancake. Makes 8.

*"Alternatively, use pre-bought ice-cream wafer cones and fill with fruit."*

# Guacca

1 Avocado, mashed **mct, ai, al, p**
¼ Medium Onion, finely diced **al**
1 Chili, finely diced **al**
½ Lemon, juiced **al**
Salt **al** and Cracked Black Pepper to taste **ac**
Place onion, chili, lemon juice, and salt in a bowl and marinade
for 30 minutes. Roughly mash avocado and fold together.
Season with cracked black pepper.

Serve with pita chips **ac** or vegetables sticks **al.**

*"This can be used as a great snack or spread."*

# Herb-Stuffed Chicken with a Mushroom Sauce

6 Chicken Thigh Fillets **al, p**
3 Slices Stale Bread **ac**
½ Small Onion, finely chopped **al**
½ Clove Garlic, finely chopped **ai**
½ Teaspoon finely chopped Sage or Mint **al**
1 Teaspoon each of finely chopped Rosemary, Thyme,
Basil, and Parsley **p, al**
2 Tablespoons Olive Oil **mct, ai**
Season to taste **al**

Blitz bread in a food processor.

In a bowl, combine crumb and rest of ingredients, mix well, and press onto thighs.

Roll up and cook in an electric skillet, on medium heat, covered, for 15 minutes each side.

Mushroom Sauce

6 Medium Mushrooms, peeled and sliced **al**
1 Tablespoon Butter **neutral**
2 Teaspoons Corn Flour **ac**
½ Cup Stock **al**
Season with Salt and Cracked Black Pepper **al**

Blend stock and corn flour together.

Cook mushrooms in a pot with butter over med/low heat, until tender; season.

Pour in liquid and boil until thickened.

Serve on a bed of Leafy Greens.

# Herbed Mini Meat Loaf Sliders with Capsicum Pear Relish

500 g Beef Mince **ac, p**
2 Slices Stale Bread **ac**
60 ml Cold Water
½ Large Onion, finely chopped **al**
½ Carrot, grated **al**
¼ Cup Frozen Peas **al**
½ Cup pureed Tomato **al, p**
1 Teaspoon each of finely chopped Rosemary, Thyme, Basil, Sage, Oregano **al**
1 Tablespoon chopped Parsley **al, p**
2 Cloves Garlic, finely chopped **ai, al**
Season to taste **al**

Combine bread with water; set aside for 15 minutes.

Mash together until mushy.

Place all ingredients (except peas), into a mixing bowl and mix together.

Fold through peas.

Shape mince into mini, flat, rectangular meat loafs and BBQ.

Serve with Capsicum Pear Relish (recipe in this book) and lettuce on small slider rolls.

> *"This is a great alternative to sausage sandwiches
> or jazz up that hamburger."*

# Home-Style Tandoori Chicken

6 Chicken Thigh Fillets **al, p**
½ Cup Yoghurt **neutral, p**
½ Small Onion, finely diced **al**
¼ Cup Lemon Juice **al**
3 Cloves Garlic, crushed **ai, al**
2 Teaspoons each of grated Ginger **ai, al** and ground Coriander **al**
1 Teaspoon each of Cumin, Chili Powder, and Salt **al**
½ Teaspoon Paprika **al**

Place the onion, garlic, ginger, and lemon juice into a food processor to make a smooth paste.

Combine the paste with the paprika, chili, coriander, cumin, salt, and yoghurt; mix together.

Place the chicken in a bowl, coat with the mixture, cover, and place in the fridge for approximately 4 hours.

Cook on the BBQ on med/low heat for approximately 6-8 minutes each side.

Serve with Indian Inspired Potatoes (recipe in this book).

# Hot Cos Salad

12 Large Cos Lettuce leaves torn into 4 **al**
3 Tablespoons Olive Oil **mct, ai**
½ Red Capsicum, sliced into matchsticks **al**
½ Medium Onion, sliced superfine **al**
2 Tablespoons Lemon Juice **al**
3 Tablespoons Feta Cheese, crumbled **ac**
Season with Salt and Cracked Black Pepper **al**

Heat oil in a pan over low heat, add capsicum, and stir for 1 minute.

Increase heat to med/high, add lettuce, and stir for 1 minute, coating all the leaves.

Remove the items.

Reduce heat to low.

Add onion and lemon juice to pan, cover, and cook for 30 seconds.

Return items back into pan; mix through.

Serve with feta and cracked black pepper.

*"This makes a fantastic lunch or dinner side dish."*

# Hot Prawns on Ribbon Vegetables

12 Green King Prawns **ac**
2 Teaspoons Salt **al**
¼ Teaspoon White Pepper **ac**
¼ Teaspoon Chili Powder **al**
Olive Oil **mct, ai**
1 Carrot and 1 Zucchini, sliced into ribbons **al**
½ Cup Bean Sprouts **al**
1 Clove Garlic, crushed **ai, al**
½ Teaspoon grated Ginger **ai, al**
Season vegetables to taste **al**

Grind salt, pepper, and chili into a fine powder.

Pat dry prawns and coat in a little olive oil; sprinkle salt mix on both sides of prawns.

Cook on char grill.

In a hot pan or wok, heat 1 tablespoon of oil; add garlic, ginger, vegetables, and seasoning.

Stir-fry for 2 minutes.

**NB**

To eat this dish, lick the outside of the prawn, then peel and eat.

*"This dish will require a finger bowl. Enjoy!"*

# Hummus Jingle Bells

½ Can Chickpeas **ac**
2 Tablespoons Lemon Juice **al**
2 Tablespoons Tahini Paste **ac**
¼ Clove Garlic, crushed **ai, al**
1 Tablespoon Olive Oil **mct, ai**
½ Teaspoon Salt **al**
¼ Teaspoon Cumin **al**
2 Tablespoons Water
24 Truss cherry tomatoes **al**
Basil Leaves to garnish **al**

In a food processor, add the tahini and lemon juice and blend until creamy, approximately 1½ minutes, occasionally scraping down the sides.

Add oil, garlic, cumin, and salt.

Process for a further 1 minute, occasionally scraping down the sides.

Drain the liquid from the chickpeas; rinse well.

Add half of the chickpeas to food processor and blend for 1 minute, scrape down the sides, and add the remaining chickpeas plus water and process for an additional 1-2 minutes.

Wash some cherry tomatoes, slice off ⅓ from the top, scoop out seeds.

Fill with hummus and top with a basil leaf. Makes approximately 24.

***"These are fun and entertaining!"***

# Indian-Inspired Potatoes

4 Medium Potatoes **ac, p**
2 Tablespoons Olive Oil **mct, ai**
1 Medium Onion, sliced **al**
1 Clove Garlic, crushed **ai, al**
½ Teaspoon Cumin **al**
1 Teaspoon Ground Coriander **al**
1 Teaspoon Yellow Mustard Seeds **al**
2 Teaspoons Curry Powder **al**
Season to taste **al**

Cut potatoes into small chunks and boil, steam, or microwave until tender.

In a nonstick pan, heat oil and add onions and garlic.

Cook until onions are soft.

Add remaining ingredients and stir until you start to smell the fragrance from the spices.

Add potatoes and gently stir to combine until heated through.

Serve with yoghurt **neutral, p** and beans **al.**

Can be accompanied by Home-style Tandoori Chicken (recipe in this book) or a nice alterative potato recipe to jazz up a weekly meal.

# Indian Stuffed Potatoes with Raita

Potato Ingredients

4 Med. Brushed Potatoes, washed **ac, p**
½ Med. Onion, finely diced **al**
2 Teaspoons Curry Powder **al**
2 Teaspoons grated Ginger **ai, al**
½ Teaspoon Brown Mustard Seeds **al**
2 Tablespoons chopped Mint **al**
1 Tablespoon finely chopped Coriander **al**
½ Cup Frozen Peas, cooked **al**
1-2 Tablespoons Olive Oil **mct, ai**
3 Tablespoons Butter **neutral**
Season to taste **al**

Prick potatoes all over with a fork and microwave on high, in an 850 watt microwave, for 9 minutes.

Remove and wrap in foil; place in a pre-heated 180º C oven for 30 minutes.

In a fry pan over med/low heat, add 1 tablespoon of olive oil to start plus the onion, curry powder, ginger, and mustard seeds.

Cook until softened, adding another tablespoon of oil if necessary.

Split potatoes ¾ way through, lengthways, scoop out flesh, and mash together with butter, onion mix, peas, coriander, and salt.

Spoon back into potato cases. Top with Raita.

Raita

1 Cup Yoghurt **neutral, p**
½ Cup diced Lebanese Cucumber **al**
Split cucumber lengthways, scoop out seeds, and finely dice.
2 Tablespoons chopped Mint **al**
Season to taste **al**

Mix all ingredients together.

# Italian Pork and Beans

750 g Pork, fat removed, cut into chunks **ac, p**
1 Extra Large Onion, cut into wedges **al**
1 Tablespoon chopped Rosemary **al**
3 Cloves Garlic, chopped **ai, al**
1 Tablespoon chopped Thyme **al**
3 Tablespoons chopped Parsley **al p,**
1 Tablespoon chopped Basil **al**
1 Teaspoon Sugar **ac**
2 Tablespoons Olive Oil **mct, ai**
1 Tin Bean Mix, drained and rinsed **ac, p**
2 x 400 g tinned Tomatoes + Juice, crushed **al, p**
Season to taste **al**

In a large pot over med/high heat, add oil and pork, season, and brown slightly.

Add garlic and herbs and combine with pork.

Add onions, tomatoes + juice, sugar, and beans; adjust seasoning.

Cover and slowly simmer for 2 hours.

Serve with yoghurt **neutral, p.**

Serves 6

*"I leave the Pork out to make this a vegetarian dish."*

# Jaeger Schnitzel with a Pickled Slaw

4 x Pork Sirloins **ac, p**
Breadcrumbs **ac**
½ Cup of Milk **ac, p**
1 Egg, beaten **al**
Plain Flour, seasoned **ac**
Olive Oil **mct, ai**

Beat the milk and egg together in a bowl to make a wash; set aside.

With a meat mallet, gently pound the pork until 5 mm thick.

Flour the pork to coat evenly, dip into the egg wash and then into the breadcrumbs.

Repeat the process with the remaining pork.

In a pan, heat olive oil and cook schnitzels until golden on both sides.

Drain on paper towel.

Garnish with parsley **al, p.**

Serve with Pickled Slaw (recipe in this book).

# Khichri

1 x 200 g tin Smoked Kippers in spring water **ac, p**
3 Cups cooked Rice **ac**
½ Onion, finely diced **al**
2 Tablespoons chopped Parsley **al, p**
1 Tablespoon Butter **neutral**
2 Medium Boiled Eggs, chopped **al**
Chili to taste **al**
Season to taste **al**

Keep rice warm.

In a small pot, melt butter on med/low heat and cook onion until soft.

Heat kippers to directions and flake.

Add all ingredients to rice and combine, gently.

Serve with lemon wedges **al.**

# Kristin's Mess

4 Egg Whites **al**
¾ Cup of Raw Sugar **ac**
1 Teaspoon Lemon Juice **al**
½ Teaspoon Vanilla Extract **ac**
Sweetened Natural Yoghurt **neutral, p**
Cherries, deseeded, and Strawberries, halved **al**
85% Dark Chocolate **mct, ac**

**Pavlova Method**

In a mortar and pestle, grind the sugar to a fine texture.

Beat egg whites until soft peaks form.

Slowly add sugar a little at a time, beating until glossy, around 7 minutes.

Beat in lemon juice and vanilla.

Line a baking tray with baking paper and spread mixture out to a 20 cm circle.

Bake at 150° C in a fan forced oven for 30 minutes and then reduce back to 120° C for a further 45 minutes.

Turn the oven off and allow the Pavlova to cool completely, with the door slightly open.

Gently break up the meringue into individual ramekins.

Dollop yoghurt and top with cherries, strawberries, and grated dark chocolate.

# Lamb, Tzatziki, and Tabbouleh Pizza

<u>Pizza</u>

4 Pita Breads **ac**
2 Cups chopped, cooked Lamb **ac, p**
2 Tomatoes, flesh removed and diced **al, p**
½ Medium Onion, finely sliced **al**
Olive Oil **mct, ai**

Brush breadswith oil, top with lamb, tomato, onion.
Bake on 200° C for 10 minutes.

Top with Tabbouleh and Tzatziki (recipes in this book).

# Lamb Vegetable Soup

1 Kg Lamb Off cuts **ac, p**
1 Large Onion, diced **al**
2 Sticks Celery with leaves, diced **ai, p**
2 Carrots, 1 grated, 1 diced **al**
1 Parsnip, ½ grated, ½ diced **al, p**
½ Swede, ¼ grated, ¼ diced **al, p**
1 Clove Garlic, crushed **ai, al**
1 Tablespoon chopped Parsley **al, p**
3-4 Sprigs of Thyme **al**
2 Litres Water
Season to taste **al**

Remove fat from lamb, place in a large boiler with water, bring to the boil, reduce heat, and simmer, covered, for 1½ hours.

Take lamb out, remove meat from bones, and refrigerate.

Strain the stock into another pot and add the remaining ingredients.

Simmer, covered, for 1 hour.

Return lamb back into pot.

For best results, place in refrigerator overnight.

The next day, skim the fat from the surface before reheating again.

*"We freeze the soup in small, single-serve containers for a quick, healthy lunch during the cooler months."*

# Lamb Yeeros with Gremolata

4 Pita Breads **ac**
4 Cups Lamb, sliced, cooked **ac, p**
8 Tablespoons Yoghurt **neutral, p**
Olive Oil **mct, ai**
Season to taste **al**

Gremolata

½ Cup finely chopped Parsley **al, p**
1 Clove Garlic, finely grated **ai, al**
Zest of 1 Large Lemon **al**
½ Tablespoon finely chopped Mint **al**
Combine all ingredients together and chop until very fine.

Method

Brush pita with oil and place in a heated pan to warm through.

Smear yoghurt all over the pita bread and sprinkle on gremolata.

Heat lamb in microwave, place on pita bread, season, and roll up.

***"This is a great lunch dish that uses up leftover lamb."***

# Lemon Chicken with Tomatoes

1 Whole Chicken, skinned and jointed **al, p**
3 Cloves Garlic, chopped **ai, al**
1 Whole Lemon Rind **al**
2 Tomatoes, split and quartered **al, p**
1 Large Onion, cut into wedges **al**
3 Tablespoons chopped Parsley **al, p**
6 Sprigs Thyme **al**
150 ml Stock **al**
Season to taste **al**

Place chicken in a casserole dish; sprinkle with garlic, parsley, and thyme.

Scatter onions and tomatoes over top.

Nestle lemon rind down in the centre.

Season and pour over stock.

Cover and bake at 180° C for 1½ hours.

# Lemon Potatoes

800 g peeled Potatoes **ac, p**
150 ml Hot Water
1 Teaspoon Stock Powder **al**
25-30 ml Lemon Juice **al**
1 Clove Garlic, sliced **ai, al**
1 Chili, sliced **ai, al**
½ Small Onion, finely sliced **al**
Olive Oil **mct, ai**

Peel potatoes and cut into chunks.

Scatter onion and garlic into baking dish, then place in potatoes.

Combine water, stock, and lemon juice, and pour into dish.

Drizzle oil over each potato and cover dish with foil.

Bake at 180º C for 1 hour.

Sprinkle with chilies **al** before serving.

*"These are a delicious, healthy alternative to chips or oily baked potatoes and go great with fish or chicken."*

# Lentil Curry

½ Cup Raw Lentils **ac**
(cook in vegetable stock as per packet directions)
1 Teaspoon each of Turmeric **al, ai** and Paprika **al**
½ Teaspoon Cumin **al**
4 Tablespoons chopped Coriander **al**
1 Teaspoon fresh Ginger **al**
2 Teaspoons Sugar **ac**
1 Large Onion, chopped **al**
2 x 400 g tins Tomatoes + Juice, crushed **al, p**
2 Cloves Garlic, crushed **ai, al**
3 Tablespoons chopped Parsley **al, p**
2 Carrots and 1 Stick Celery, diced **ai, p, al**
4 Tablespoons Olive Oil **mct, ai**
Chili to taste **al**
Season to taste **al**

In a large pot over med/low heat, add 1 tablespoon of oil and cook onion, garlic, celery, carrot, and chili until tender; remove from pan and set aside.

Scatter turmeric, cumin, ginger, and paprika over top, and stir to coat all the vegetables.

Add tomatoes, sugar, coriander, and parsley.

Season and slowly simmer, covered, for 1½ hours.

Serve with yoghurt **neutral, p** and rice or cous cous and greens.

# Lo-Carb Cannelloni

## Ingredients Filling

500 g Beef Mince **ac, p**
1 x 200 g Frozen Spinach, chopped and squeezed dry **al, p** or
400 g Fresh Spinach Leaves, boiled for 10 minutes, squeezed dry, and chopped
1 Small Onion, finely diced **al**
1 Clove Garlic, crushed **ai, al**
2 Tablespoons chopped Parsley **al, p**
3 Tablespoons grated Parmesan Cheese **ac**
1 Teaspoon Ground Nutmeg **al**
½ Cup Fresh Breadcrumbs **ac**
2 Eggs, beaten **al**
2 Teaspoons Olive Oil **mct, ai**
Season with Salt **al** and Cracked Black Pepper **ac**

In a pan over med/low heat, add olive oil, onion, and garlic; cook until softened; and remove.

Increase heat to high and cook mince until just brown, drain fat, and stir through onion, garlic, spinach, parsley, nutmeg, Parmesan cheese, breadcrumbs, and seasoning.

Add the eggs, mix thoroughly, remove, and cool.

## Napolitano Sauce

1 Small Onion, finely diced **al**
3 Cloves Garlic, crushed **ai, al**
2 Teaspoons finely chopped Basil **al**
1 Tablespoon chopped Parsley **al, p**
2 Teaspoons Sugar **ac**
2 Teaspoons Olive Oil **mct, ai**
2 x 400 g Tin Tomatoes + Juice crushed **al, p**
Season to taste **al**

In a saucepan over med/low heat, add olive oil, onion, and garlic; cook until softened. Add tomatoes, parsley, basil, sugar, and seasoning. Cover and simmer for 20 minutes, remove lid, and continue to cook until sauce has reduced and thickened. Remove and cool.

Cannelloni Batter

1 Cup Plain Flour **ac**, Pinch Salt **al**, 1 Egg **al**, 1 Cup Milk **ac, p**
(Beat together)

Pre-heat a frying pan over med-high heat; coat pan with a little butter.

Pour ¼ cup of batter into the centre and swirl around to distribute evenly. When cooked on one side, flip, cook the other side, remove, and stack. Makes 8 crepes.

Assembly

Divide filling between crepes and roll up. Place into a 3-litre baking dish, spoon sauce over top, and bake at 250º C for 15 minutes.

Garnish with parsley **al, p.**

# Lunchtime Special

<u>Spinach Delight</u>

2 Cups, packed, shredded Spinach **al, p**
1 Eye of Bacon, diced **ac**
¼ Medium Onion, diced **al**
½ Clove Garlic, crushed **ai, al**
1 Teaspoon Thyme **al**
1 Tablespoon Olive Oil **mct, ai**
1 Tablespoon Feta Cheese, crumbled **ac**
Season to taste **al**

Method

In a frying pan over medium heat add oil, onion, garlic and bacon, fry until onion softens.

Add thyme, spinach and seasoning, cooking for a further 5 minutes, stirring regularly.

Place into a crusty roll and top with feta cheese.

<u>Egg and Lettuce Treat</u>

1 Egg, boiled and mashed **al**
1 Tablespoon grated Parmesan Cheese **ac**
½ Tablespoon chopped Parsley **al, p**
4 Slices Avocado **mct, al, ai, p**
Shredded Lettuce **al**
Season to taste **al**

Mix together egg, parmesan cheese, parsley and season.

On a crusty roll place the lettuce and avocado then top with the egg mixture.

# Marinated BBQ Vegetables

2 Medium Zucchini **al**
1 Small Eggplant **al**
1 Red Capsicum **al**
1 Large Red Onion **al**
2 Cloves Garlic, crushed **al, ai**
1 Tablespoon, finely chopped Basil **al**
2 Teaspoons, finely chopped Thyme **al**
3 Tablespoons Olive Oil **mct, ai**
2½ Tablespoons Brown Vinegar **ac**
½ Teaspoon Sugar **ac**
½ Teaspoon Salt **al**

Slice zucchini diagonally into 1 cm thick slices.

Slice eggplant into 1 cm thick rings, then cut into quarters.

Split capsicum into quarters lengthways and slice diagonally into 3-4 pieces. Cut onion into 8 wedges.

In a bowl blend together, olive oil, garlic, basil, thyme, vinegar, sugar and salt.

Toss through vegetables and marinate for 1 hour.

Cook on a pre-heated BBQ plate, on medium heat, for 10-12 minutes, until tender and slightly charred.

*"We have this with tuna steaks."*

# Meatzza

4 Whole meal Pita Breads **ac**

125 g Beef Mince **ac, p**

Garlic Oil

1 Clove Garlic, crushed **ai, al**

Parmesan Cheese to sprinkle over top **ac**

Basil leaves to garnish **al**

2 Tablespoons Olive Oil **mct, ai**

Combine and infuse for 2 hours

Tomato Sauce

1 x 400 g tin Tomatoes + Juice, crushed **al, p**

1 Clove Garlic, crushed **ai, al**

1 Teaspoon each of chopped Thyme, Basil, Marjoram **al**

1 Teaspoon Sugar **ac**

Chili to taste **al**

Season to taste **al**

Place all ingredients in a covered pot and simmer for 20 minutes.

Remove lid and cook until sauce is reduced and thickened.

Brush garlic oil over base of pizza.

Place on small pinches of raw mince evenly around pizza.

Randomly scatter sauce and bake at 250º C for 5-10 minutes.

Sprinkle with cheese and garnish with basil.

Serve with lemon **al** and yoghurt **neutral, p.**

*"We wanted to create an easy alternative to Italian Meatballs in Tomato Sauce with Garlic Bread, so we combined the lot and put it onto a Pizza. Ben named it!"*

# Mediterranean Medley

500 g Lamb Mince **ac, p**
2 Teaspoons chopped Basil **al**
2 Eggplants **al**
2 Teaspoons chopped Thyme **al**
½ Cup crumbled Feta Cheese **ac**
1 Teaspoon Curry Powder **al**
½ Medium Onion, diced **al**
1 Teaspoon Sugar **ac**
1 Clove Garlic, crushed **ai, al**
2 Teaspoons Olive Oil **mct, ai**
1 x 400 g Tin Tomatoes + Juice, crushed **al, p**
Season to taste **al**

In a pan over med/low heat add oil, onion, and garlic; cook until soft; and remove.

Increase heat to high add mince, brown, and drain excess oil.

Return onion and garlic, stir in curry powder and add tomatoes, basil, thyme, sugar, and seasoning.

Cover and simmer for 1½ hours, remove lid, and reduce for 20-30 minutes.

In the meantime, slice eggplant lengthways into 4 slices and sprinkle with salt on both sides, leave for 30 minutes, wash salt off, and pat dry.

Cook both sides in an oiled pan, on medium.

When the eggplant is cooked, spoon mixture over the top and sprinkle with feta cheese.

# Mini Chicken Meatball and Sweet Corn Soup

<u>Stock Ingredients</u>

1 Chicken Frame from a 2 kg Chicken **al, p**
1 Litre Water
1 Medium Onion, halved, 1 Carrot, peeled, 1 Stick Celery **al, p**
Seasoning **al**

Place all ingredients in a large stock pot, bring to the boil, and then simmer covered for 1½ hours, then strain.

| <u>Ingredients</u> | <u>Mini Chicken Meatballs</u> |
|---|---|
| 1 Medium Onion, finely diced **al** | 250 g Chicken Mince **al, p** |
| 1 Cup pureed Corn Kernels **al** | 1 Tablespoon Bread Crumbs **ac** |
| 1 Tablespoon Olive Oil **mct, ai** | Season to taste **al** |
| 2 Eggs, beaten **al** | |
| Shallots finely sliced **al** | |

Combine chicken mince, breadcrumbs, and seasoning.

With wet hands, roll into mini meatballs. Makes approximately 40-45.

Put olive oil in a pot over med/low heat and cook onion until soft, not allowing any colour to form.

Pour in stock and corn and bring to a simmer, season, and drop in the mini chicken meatballs, 1 by 1.

Cover and simmer, gently, for 10 minutes.

Remove from heat and stir in beaten eggs. Garnish with shallots **al.**

# Moroccan Roasted Vegetables

500 g Potato **ac, p**
400 g Sweet Potato **ai, al, p**
1 Red Onion **al**
2 Parsnips **al, p**
2 Carrots **al**
3-4 Tablespoons Olive Oil **mct, ai**
1 Teaspoon each of Ground Cumin, Ground Coriander, Ground Cinnamon and Paprika **al**
½ Teaspoon Ground Turmeric **al**
Season to taste **al**

Peel potatoes and cut into equal size pieces.

Peel onion and cut into 8 wedges.

Peel parsnips and carrots and cut into ¼ lengthways.

Blend together spices, seasoning and olive oil.

Toss vegetables in oil and spice mix.

Bake in a tray for 1½ hours at 180º C or until tender.

Garnish with fresh coriander. **al.**

# Nachos with Avocado Salsa

1 Avocado, diced **mct, al, ai, p**
1 Small Tomato, finely diced **al**
¼ Medium Onion, finely diced **al**
¼ Red Capsicum, finely diced **al**
2 Tablespoons finely chopped Parsley **al, p**
½ Chili, finely diced **al**
1 Tablespoon Olive Oil **mct, ai**
¼ Large Lemon, juiced **al**
Season with Salt **al** and Cracked Black Pepper **ac**
2 Tablespoons grated Tasty Cheese **ac**
1 x Packet 5-7 Pita Breads **ac**

Gently combine all ingredients together except the cheese.

Place pita breads in a hot oven, approximately 210º C, for 5-10 minutes or until slightly golden and crunchy.

Cut up into bite-size chips.

Sprinkle cheese over pita chips and place under a hot grill until the cheese has melted, being careful not to burn them.

# Pickled Slaw

2-3 Large Cabbage leaves, cut into 1 cm strips **al**
1 Small Onion, sliced into ½ cm rings **al**
½ Stick Celery, sliced into ½ cm pieces **al, ai,**
1 Small Carrot, sliced into ½ cm rings **al**
¼ Red Capsicum, halved and sliced into ½ cm strips **al**
2-Litre Jar

Pickling Mixture

2½ Cups White Vinegar **ac**
2½ Cups Hot Water
3 Tablespoons Sugar **ac**
4 Teaspoons Yellow Mustard Seeds **al**
2 Teaspoons Salt **al**
12 Black Pepper Corns **ac**
1 Teaspoon Dried Chili **al**
2 Cloves Garlic, sliced **ai, al**
4 Teaspoons Dill Seeds **al**
8 Thick Parsley Stems **al, p**

In a saucepan, combine the pickling mixture ingredients, bring to the boil, reduce heat, and simmer for 5 minutes.

Place vegetables into a large, hot, sterilised jar and pour over the mixture.

Seal at once and allow to cool, then refrigerate.

## Poached Pears with Almond Walnut Crumble

4 Pears **al, p**
1 Cup Water
1 Tablespoon Butter **neutral**
1 Tablespoon Honey **al**
2 Tablespoons Lemon Juice **al**
¼ Cup Sugar **ac**
⅓ Cup crushed Walnuts **mct, ai, ac**
⅓ Cup crushed Almonds **mct, al, p**
Cinnamon to serve **al**

Peel, split, and decore pears.

Bring water, lemon juice, butter, sugar, and honey to the boil; add pears, core side down. Reduce heat, cover, and simmer for 15-20 minutes or until pears are tender.

Place combined nuts on a tray and bake at 180° C for 3-5 minutes. Set aside.

Place nuts in the bottom of a serving bowl, place in pear, spoon syrup over top, and dust with cinnamon.

# Prawn Noodle Salad

12 Large, cooked Prawns, peeled **ac, p**
100 g Flat Rice Noodles **ac**
2 Teaspoons Sesame Oil **ac**
2 Chilies, finely sliced **al**
¼ Red Onion, finely sliced **al**
¼ Red Capsicum **al**
Salt to taste **al**

Prepare noodles to packet instructions and drain well.

Split capsicum lengthways and slice a quarter into long, thin strips.

Combine all ingredients in a bowl and mix well to coat noodles.

Garnish with coriander **al.**

# Prawn Pasta Carbonara

12 Green Prawns, peeled and deveined **ac**
250 g Dry Spaghetti **ac**
2 Eggs **al**
¼ Cup Parmesan Cheese, grated **ac**
¼ Medium Onion, finely diced **al**
1 Clove Garlic, crushed **ai, al**
1 Chili, finely diced **al**
1 Cup Broccoli Florets **ai, al**
2 Tablespoons chopped Parsley **al, p**
2 Tablespoons Olive Oil **mct, ai**
Pinch of Salt **al**
Cracked Black Pepper **ac**

Cook broccoli until just tender, cover, and set aside to keep warm.

Beat eggs and Parmesan cheese together and set aside.

Start cooking spaghetti in a large pot of boiling, salted water.

Place a pan on med/low heat; add olive oil, onion, garlic, chili, and season with a pinch of salt. Cook until softened.

Increase heat to med, add prawns, and cook for 2 minutes each side.

When spaghetti is al dente, drain briefly and add the prawns, toss together, and set aside to cool slightly, approximately 2 minutes. This stops the eggs scrambling.

Pour over egg and cheese mixture, toss through until cheese is melted, add broccoli.

Serve topped with cracked black pepper and parsley.

# Quick Tomato Soup

1 Medium Onion, finely chopped **al**
2 Cloves Garlic, crushed **ai, al**
4 Teaspoons Sugar **ac**
2 Tablespoons Butter **neutral**
4 x 400 g Tinned Tomatoes + Juice **al, p**
Season to taste **al**

In a saucepan, on medium heat, melt butter; add onion, garlic, and sugar; and cook until onion is caramel in colour.

Add tomatoes, seasoning, and bring to the boil.

Cover and simmer for 30 minutes.

Blitz to serve.

Serving suggestions include cracked black pepper **ac**, basil **al**, and yoghurt **neutral, p.**

# Salmon Pasta Salad

1 x 200-250 g Atlantic Salmon Fillet, cooked,
cooled, and flaked **ai, al, p**
250 g Dry Penne Pasta **ac**
1 packed Cup of finely shredded Lettuce **al**
1 Tomato, diced **al**
¼ Lebanese Cucumber, split and finely sliced **al**
¼ Red Capsicum, finely sliced **al**
½ Stick Celery, finely sliced **ai, al, p**
½ Small Onion, finely sliced **al**
3 Tablespoons chopped Parsley **al, p**
Brown Malt Vinegar to taste **ac**
Season to taste **al**

Cook pasta in salted boiling water, drain and rinse under cold water, then drain well.

Divide all ingredients between two plates, layering with pasta, lettuce, tomato, cucumber, capsicum, celery, onion, salmon, and parsley.

Alternatively, toss all ingredients together.

Season and drizzle with brown vinegar.

# Salsa Bonné Bouché

1 Large Tomato, finely chopped **al**
1 Shallot or ¼ Small Onion, finely chopped **al**
½ Tablespoon each of Celery and Parsley, finely chopped **al, p, ai**
1 Tablespoon Red Capsicum, finely chopped **al**
½ Clove Garlic, finely chopped **ai, al**
1 Teaspoon each of Basil and Chili, finely chopped **al**
1 Teaspoon Olive Oil **mct, ai**
Juice of ¼ Lemon **al**
Salt **al** and Cracked Black Pepper **ac**

Combine all ingredients in a bowl and mix well.

Serve with water crackers or pita chips.

To make the Bonné Bouché, leave the salsa overnight and drain off the liquid.

Pour the drained liquid into shot glasses and pop in a peeled, cooked prawn.

*"This is a great appetiser for parties."*

# Sautéed Mustard Greens

450 g Zucchini, halved and sliced **al**
250 g Green Beans, topped and tailed **al**
6 Large Shallots, split lengthways **al**
2 Cloves Garlic, finely chopped **ai, al**
2 Tablespoons Butter **neutral**
2 Teaspoons Brown Mustard Seeds **al**
Season with Salt **al** and Cracked Black Pepper **ac**

In a pan over medium heat, melt 1 tablespoon butter, add beans, and cook for 5 minutes.

Add another tablespoon of butter; add zucchini, garlic, and seasoning; and cook until the zucchini just starts to soften, approximately 5 minutes.

Add mustard seeds and shallots and continue cooking for a further 5 minutes or until the vegetables reach a desired texture.

*"This is a lovely side dish for any meat or white fish."*

# Savoury Chicken Pie

250 g Chicken Thighs **al, p**
1½ Tablespoons seasoned Flour **ac**
3 Tablespoons Olive Oil **mct, ai**
½ Clove Garlic, crushed **ai, al**
¼ Red Capsicum, diced **al**
½ Carrot and ½ Stick Celery, diced **ai, p, al**
½ x 400 g Tinned Tomatoes + Juice, crushed **al, p**
½ Cup Stock **al**
1½ Tablespoons chopped Parsley **al, p**
Salt **al** and Cracked Black Pepper **ac**
1 Tablespoon Corn Flour **ac**

Pastry

¼ Cup Plain Flour **ac**
½ Medium Onion, diced **al**
¼ Cup Self-Raising Flour **ac**
½ Tablespoon Butter **neutral**
2-3 Tablespoons Cold Water

In a pot, add oil; cook onion, garlic, capsicum, carrot, and celery until tender; remove from pan. Dust chicken in flour, brown both sides, and return cooked vegetables.

Add tomatoes, stock, parsley, and season. Simmer covered for 1½ hours. Remove chicken and shred.

Mix corn flour in a little water, stir, and cook until thickened.

Return chicken. Cool mixture. Place mixture into ramekin dishes.

<u>Pastry</u>

Sift both flours together, add butter, and rub through, until crumbly.

Add water, bring together with a knife, and roll out, thinly, to cover top of pies.

Bake at 180° C 30-40 minutes.

Serves 2

# Seared Tuna Steak on a Vinegar Broccoli Mash

4 Tuna Steaks **al, p**
500 g peeled Potatoes **ac, p**
250 g Broccoli heads **ai, al**
100 ml Brown Vinegar **ac**
Season to taste **al**

Boil, steam, or microwave potatoes and broccoli separately.

Mash together with the brown vinegar and seasoning.

Sear tuna on a BBQ or griddle pan until liking.

Serve the tuna on a bed of the vinegar mash.

# Singapore Noodles

12 Peeled Cooked King Prawns **ac**
100 g Dry Rice Noodles **ac**
(Prepared to packet instructions and drained well)
1 Egg **al**
2 Tablespoons Frozen Peas **al**
½ Large Onion, sliced **al**
½ Red Capsicum, sliced **al**
1 Green Shallot, sliced **al**
½ Teaspoon grated Ginger **ai, al**
½ Tablespoon Curry Powder **al**
1 Tablespoon Oil **mct, ai**
¼ Teaspoon Sesame Oil **ac**
30 ml Vegetable Stock **al**
Season to taste **al**

Blend together the stock, sesame oil, and curry powder and set aside.

In a wok, over high heat, add oil and the egg and scramble until it just turns; add the onion, capsicum, and ginger; and stir-fry for 1½-2 minutes.

Add the noodles, prawns, peas, and salt, blending the ingredients together. Stir-fry for 1 minute.

Toss through shallots and serve.

Serves 2

# Smoked Nicoise Cups

12 Cos Lettuce Leaves **al**
200 g Potato, peeled **ac, p**
1 x 125 g Tin Smoked Tuna in Olive Oil,
(drained and shredded) **mct, p**
80 g Snow Peas **al**
½ Medium Onion, finely diced **al**
1 Tomato, diced **al, p**
2 Boiled Eggs, diced **al**
2 Tablespoons chopped Parsley **al, p**
Season with Salt **al** and Cracked Black Pepper **ac**

Microwave, boil, or steam potatoes until tender, cool, and cut into 1 cm cubes.

Blanch snow peas for 2 minutes and plunge into cold water.

Dry and slice diagonally into 1 cm strips.

Toss all ingredients together with vinaigrette and spoon into lettuce cups.

Serves 2

Dijon Vinaigrette (Blend all ingredients together)

2 Tablespoons White Vinegar **ac**
1 Teaspoon each of Lemon Juice **al,** sugar **ac,** and olive oil **mct, ai**
½ Teaspoon Dijon Mustard **ac**
Season to taste **al**

***"This is an alternative to using bread."***

## Southern Herbed Chicken on Bubble 'n' Squeak Mash with Tomato and Onion Bake

500 g Chicken Thigh Fillets or Breasts **al, p**
1 CupMilk **ac, p**
½ Cup Plain Flour **ac**
1 Teaspoon each of finely chopped Rosemary, Thyme, Mint, Sage, Marjoram **al**
1 Tablespoon finely chopped Parsley **al, p**
Season to taste **al**

Combine rosemary, thyme, mint, sage, marjoram, and parsley into seasoned flour.

Pat the chicken dry, dip in milk, and press into flour, coating well.

**NB**

Do not flour the chicken too far in advance (no more than 30 minutes) because the flour will go soggy.

Pan-fry the chicken until golden.

Serve with Bubble 'n' Squeak Mash and Tomato and Onion Bake (recipes in this book).

# Spaghetti Napolitano with Poached Egg

500 g Dry Spaghetti **ac**
1 Rash Bacon, diced **ac, p**
1 Small Onion, finely diced **al**
3 Cloves Garlic, finely chopped **ai, al**
1 Teaspoon Thyme **al**
2 Teaspoons chopped Basil **al**
1 Tablespoon chopped Parsley **al, p**
2 Teaspoons Sugar **ac**
2 x 400 g Tinned Tomatoes + Juice, crushed **al, p**
2 Teaspoons Olive Oil **mct, ai**
4 Eggs **al**
Parmesan Cheese to garnish **ac**
Chili to taste **al**
Season to taste **al**

In a pot, add oil, onion, bacon, and garlic; cook over med/low heat until soft.

Add tomatoes, sugar, basil, and parsley and bring to the simmer.

Season, cover, and cook for 20 minutes.

Uncover and continue to cook until the sauce has reduced and thickened.

Cook pasta to packet directions while poaching the eggs.

Serve with poached egg, chili, and Parmesan cheese.

> *"We make the Napolitano sauce in advance and keep it in the freezer; this makes it a quick and easy nutritious meal for Sunday night."*

# Spicy Rice Pilaf

3 Cups Cooked Rice **ac**
½ Medium Onion, finely diced **al**
¼ Cup Peas **al**
¼ Cup each of Carrot and Celery, finely diced **al, p**
1 Teaspoon Curry Powder **ac**
1 Tablespoon Olive Oil **mct, ai**
Season to taste **al**

In a pan, over med/low heat, add oil, onion, carrot, celery, and seasoning, and cook until tender.

Add rice and sprinkle with curry powder; combine.

Toss through the peas and cook until tender.

Serve with lemon **al**

**NB**

For added protein, fibre, and anthocyanins, we add a tin of black beans.

*"This can be eaten alone as a meal or accompanied with meat, chicken, or fish."*

# Spicy Stuffed Pumpkin

1 Butternut Pumpkin **al, p**
1 Cup Cooked Rice **ac**
1 Tablespoon Butter **neutral**
1½ Medium Onions, finely diced **al**
2 Tablespoons Tomato Flesh, diced **al, p**
1 Teaspoon each of Cumin, grated Ginger, Coriander, Turmeric **al, ai**
1 Clove Garlic, crushed **ai, al**
Season to taste **al**

Split pumpkin lengthways; scoop out seeds and membrane on both ends to form a cavity.

Place butter in a pan, over med/low heat, with onion and garlic; cook until tender.

Add ginger, spices, and seasoning, cooking for a further 2 minutes.

Set mixture aside to cool. Fold in with the rice and tomato.

Season pumpkin cavity prior to stuffing.

Stuff the pumpkin halves with rice mixture.

Place on a baking dish, cover with foil, and bake at 180º C for

1½ - 1¾ hours.

# Spring Picnic Slice

4 Eyes Bacon, diced **ac, p**
6 Eggs **al**
½ Cup Plain Flour **ac**
2 Zucchini, grated **al**
2 Carrots, peeled and grated **al**
1 Onion, finely diced **al**
½ Cup Fresh Corn Kernels **al**
½ Cup Peas **al**
¼ Cup chopped Parsley **al, p**
¼ Cup grated Parmesan Cheese **ac**
Season to taste **al**
Butter **neutral**

Grease a 2-litre baking dish with butter.

Beat eggs and flour together until smooth, add remaining ingredients, (except the cheese), season, and mix together well.

Pour into baking dish, sprinkle with the cheese, and bake at 180º C for 40-45 minutes.

May be eaten hot or cold.

*"This is wonderful for school lunches and picnics."*

# Spring Salad

1 Cup cooked, Fresh Corn Kernels, cooled **al**
1 x 420 g Tin Bean Mix, drained and rinsed **ac, p**
½ Cup Frozen Peas **al**
½ Medium Onion, finely diced **al**
¼ Red Capsicum, diced **al**
1 Stick Celery, diced **al, ai**
1 Tablespoon each of finely chopped Coriander and Mint **al**
Season to taste **al**

Boil peas until tender and plunge into cold water; drain.

Combine all ingredients, pour over dressing, and mix together.

Dressing

1 Tablespoon Olive Oil **mct, ai**
½ Clove Garlic, crushed **al, ai**
2 Tablespoons Lemon Juice **al**
Season to taste **al**
1 Teaspoon Sugar **ac**
1 Teaspoon Mustard Powder **al**
½ Teaspoon finely diced Chili **al**
Whisk all ingredients together.

*"This salad is very refreshing on a hot summer's night."*

# Stir-Fried Vegetables

500 g Assorted Vegetables of Choice **al**
Season to taste **al**
Olive Oil **mct, ai**

<u>Sauce</u>

1 Cup Stock **al**
1 Tablespoon Sesame Oil **ac**
1 Tablespoon Corn Flour **ac**

Combine all ingredients and set aside.

Heat wok or fry pan, add oil and vegetables, season, and stir-fry.

Stir through sauce until heated through.

This basic recipe can be used with many other recipes as an alternative to rice and pasta and is used with Stuffed Steamed Capsicums (recipe in this book).

# Stockman's Pepper Stew

500-750 g Chuck Steak **ac, p**
1 Medium Onion, diced **al**
2 Carrots and 2 Celery sticks, diced **al, p**
2 Cloves Garlic, crushed **ai, al**
½ Parsnip, diced **al, p**
3 Tablespoons Tomato Paste **al, p**
¼ Swede, diced **al, p**
3 Tablespoons Plain Flour, seasoned **ac**
3 Tablespoons chopped Parsley **al, p**
1 Cup Stock **al**
5 Tablespoons Olive Oil **mct, ai**
Salt **al** and Cracked Black Pepper **ac**

In a large pot over med/low heat, add 1 tablespoon oil, vegetables, and garlic; cook until onion is tender.

Remove from pot and set aside.

Remove the fat from the steak and cut into 3 cm cubes.

Coat steak with seasoned flour.

Increase the heat to medium, add 4 tablespoons oil, and cook meat until slightly brown.

Return the vegetables to the pot along with the stock, tomato paste, and parsley.

Season well with salt and 36 grinds of cracked black pepper; stir through.

Cover and gently simmer for 2½ - 3 hours, stirring occasionally.

Serves 6

***"This is real man's food!"***

# Stuffed Steamed Capsicums

500 g Beef Mince **ac, p**
1 Clove Garlic, crushed **ai, al**
2 Red Capsicums **al**
1 Teaspoon grated Ginger **ai, al**
2 Slices Stale Bread **ac**
1 Chili, finely diced **al**
60 ml Cold Water
1 Teaspoon Sesame Oil **ac**
½ Cup Cooked Cabbage **al**
1 Teaspoon Olive Oil **mct, ai**
1 Cup Stock **al**
1 Onion, finely diced **al**
Season to taste **al**

Place bread in a bowl with the water and set aside for 15 minutes.

Squeeze water out of cabbage. Set aside.

Slice capsicums lengthways, remove seeds, leave in stalk.

Mash bread with hand until mushy.

Combine all ingredients, except the stock, and pack capsicums with mixture.

In a large pot, bring stock to the boil, place in capsicums, cover, and simmer for 20-30 minutes.

Serve on top of Stir-Fried Vegetables (recipe in this book).

# Sunset Spritzer

5 Mint Leaves **al**
Juice of 1 tin of Sliced Pineapple **al, p**
Juice of ½ Lemon **al**
1½ Passion Fruit **al**
Ice Cubes
Mineral Water **al**

Place all ingredients into a drinking jar and stir.

Fill with mineral water to taste.

*"I enjoy drinking this after a long day at work,*
*watching the summer sun go down."*

## Surf 'n' Turf with Lemon Potatoes and Peas

4 Salmon Fillets **mct, ai, p**
6 Eyes of Bacon, thinly sliced **ac, p**
2 Cups Peas **al**

On a BBQ or in a frying pan, cook salmon and bacon strips.

Boil, steam, or microwave peas until tender.

Place fish on top of peas, top fish with bacon, and drizzle with olive oil.

Plate with Lemon Potatoes with juice (recipe in this book).

# Tabbouleh and Tzatziki

## Tabbouleh

½ Cup Cous Cous **ac**
½ Cup Boiling Water
½ Medium Onion, finely diced **al**
¾ Cup, finely chopped Parsley **al, p**
2 Tablespoons, finely chopped Mint **al**
2½ Tablespoons Olive Oil **mct, ai**
¼ Cup Lemon Juice **al**
Salt **al**
Cracked Black Pepper **ac**

In a bowl drizzle ½ tablespoon oil over cous cous.

Pour over boiling water. Cover and let stand for 2 minutes. Uncover and rake with a fork to fluff up. Refrigerate to cool.

Mix together with all of the other ingredients.

## Tzatziki

1 Cup Yoghurt **neutral, p**
1 Clove Garlic, crushed **ai, al**
2 Teaspoons Lemon Juice **al**
¼ Cup Cucumber **al**

Split cucumber lengthways, scoop out seeds, and finely dice.

Mix all ingredients together.

# Thai Crab Appetiser

Fresh Crab Meat, shredded **al**
Finely sliced, Chili **al**
Finely chopped, Shallots **al**
Finely chopped, Coriander Leaves **al**
Lemon **al**
Salt to taste **al**

Place crab meat into spoons and sprinkle with chili, shallots, and coriander.

Season to taste and squeeze over lemon juice.

# Thai Tuna Cakes and Salad

500 g Peeled Potatoes, boiled, mashed and cooled **ac, p**
1 x 185 g Tin Tuna, drained and flaked **ac, p**
½ Small Onion, finely diced **al**
2 Teaspoons Fresh Sage or Mint **al**
½ Tablespoon Lemon Juice + ¼ Teaspoon Lemon Zest **al**
2 Tablespoons chopped Parsley **al, p**
1 Chili, finely diced **al**
1 Egg **al**
¼ Cup Breadcrumbs **ac**
Season to taste **al**
Olive Oil for frying **mct, ai**

Add tuna, onion, sage/mint, lemon juice + zest, parsley, chili, egg, and seasoning to mashed potatoes.

Refrigerate until cold.

Form into 8 equal patties and crumb. Shallow-fry until golden.

**Salad Pictured**
1 Small Onion **al**
½ Telegraph Cucumber **al**
½ Red Capsicum **al**
1 Cup Bean Sprouts **al**

**Dressing**
4 Tablespoons Olive Oil **mct, ai**
½ Teaspoon Salt **ac**
2 Tablespoons each of
Lemon Juice **al** and White Vinegar **ac**
4 Teaspoons each of chopped
Coriander & Ground Ginger
2 Teaspoon chopped Mint
1 Teaspoon chopped Chili **al**
1 Tablespoon Sugar **ac**

Whisk all ingredients together.

# Tomato and Onion Bake

2 Large Tomatoes, chopped **al, p**
½ Large Onion, chopped **al**
2 Slices Bread, roughly torn **ac**
1 Tablespoon Olive Oil **mct, ai**
Cracked Black Pepper **al**
Season to taste **al**

Place tomatoes, onion, and seasoning in a baking dish; toss together.

Mix bread and oil together in a separate bowl and place on top of tomato mixture.

Bake at 160° C for 50-60 minutes or until golden.

**NB**

You can add depth of flavour to this dish by adding fresh complimentary herbs, such as oregano, basil, thyme, rosemary and parsley. You can add one or two of the above list; the choice is up to you because they all go well with tomatoes, or you can leave it nice and simple.

*"This dish always accompanies a baked dinner in our house."*

# Trail Mix

4 x Chunks of Fresh Coconut **al**
4 x Dates **al, p**
6 x Almonds **mct, al, p**
6 x Walnuts **mct, al, ai**

Slice dates, almonds, and walnuts into pieces.

Divide mixture into two separate containers, one for morning tea and one for afternoon tea or snack time.

*"I find this gives me a sugar and energy hit in between meals; this recipe replaces muesli bars."*

# Turmeric Chicken with Cauliflower Cous Cous and Roasted Almonds

1 Whole Chicken, skinned and jointed **al, p**
1 Medium Onion, sliced **al**
2 Carrots, sliced into thick rings **al**
1 Celery stick, chopped **al, p**
1 Clove Garlic, chopped **ai, al**
1 Teaspoon Turmeric **ai, al**
1 Teaspoon Dry Marjoram **al**
3 Tablespoons chopped Parsley **al, p**
3 Tablespoons Plain Flour, seasoned **ac**
1 Cup Stock **al**
Season to taste **al**

Flour chicken and place in a casserole dish with lid.

Sprinkle with onion, garlic, celery, carrot, turmeric, marjoram, parsley, and seasoning.

Pour over stock.

Bake at 180º C for 1½ hours.

Serve with Cauliflower Cous Cous and Roasted Almonds

(recipe in this book).

# Turmeric Fish with Hot Cos Salad and Potato Boulders

700 g White Fish **al, p**
½ Cup Plain Flour **ac**
1 Teaspoon Turmeric **ai, al**
Milk for coating **ac**
6 Potatoes, peeled and thickly sliced **ac, p**
Olive Oil for frying **mct, ai**
Season to taste **al**

Shallow-fry the potatoes for 10 minutes each side and place in an oven to keep warm.

In a tray, mix flour, seasoning, turmeric.

Pat fish dry, dip in milk, and press into flour, coating well.

**NB**

Do not flour fish too far in advance (no more than 30 minutes) because the flour will go soggy.

Pan-fry fish until cooked, between 4-6 minutes each side, depending on thickness.

Serve with Hot Cos Salad (recipe in this book).

*"This is our take on fish, chips, and salad during the colder months."*

# Vegetable Frittata

500 g peeled Sweet Potato, microwave until tender and
slice into 1-cm-thick pieces **ai, al, p**
1 Tablespoon Olive Oil **mct, ai**
2 Cloves Garlic, crushed **ai, al**
1 Small Onion, chopped **al**
1 Small Red Capsicum, chopped **al**
¼ Cup chopped Parsley **al, p**
6 Eggs, lightly beaten with 2 Tablespoons water **al**
¼ Cup grated Parmesan Cheese **ac**
Season to taste **al**

Heat oil in a large, nonstick fry pan over medium heat.

Add garlic, onion, and capsicum; cook for 3 minutes.

Spread evenly over pan.

Place sweet potato in a single layer and sprinkle with parsley.

Pour seasoned eggs over top and add Parmesan cheese.

Cook for 15 minutes.

Place pan under a hot grill to finish the eggs and lightly brown.

***"Can be served cold for lunch or picnics."***

# Vegetable Spaghetti Omelette

200 g Dry Spaghetti, cooked **ac**
1 Small Onion, ½ Red Capsicum, and 1 Small Tomato, diced **al, p**
4 Mushrooms, sliced **al**
3 Tablespoons chopped Parsley **al, p**
½ Cup Feta Cheese, crumbled **ac**
2 Tablespoons Olive Oil **mct, ai**
6 Eggs **al**
2 Tablespoons Water
Season with Salt **al** and Cracked Black Pepper **ac**

Combine eggs, water, and seasoning and set aside.

Add oil to a nonstick pan, over medium heat, and cook onion and capsicum until soft; add spaghetti and combine.

Spread mixture evenly over pan and layer with mushrooms.

Scatter tomato, parsley, and feta cheese over top.

Pour over egg mixture, cover with lid, and cook for 10-15 minutes.

Uncover and brown under the grill.

*"This recipe is great for using up leftover spaghetti for a quick meal."*

# Waldorf Salad with Chicken

1 Cup cooked, shredded Chicken **al, p**
1 Red and 1 Green Apple **al, p**
2 Sticks Celery, sliced **al, ai**
½ Cup finely sliced Fennel **al, ai, p**
¼ Cup Walnut pieces **mct, ai**
1 Tablespoon Lemon Juice **al**

Quarter apples. decore, and cut into small pieces.

Place into a bowl and toss through lemon juice.

Add celery, fennel, walnuts, and chicken, mix together.

Pour dressing over top and combine well.

Dressing

½ Cup Yoghurt **neutral, p**
½ Teaspoon Honey **al**
¼ Teaspoon Curry Powder **al**
Good pinch of Salt **al**

Combine all ingredients and set aside.

Serves 2

*"This is a new twist on an old recipe."*

# Zesty Stuffed Mushrooms on Garlic Cabbage

2 Large Field Mushrooms **al**
½ Teaspoon Lemon Zest **al**
¼ Small Onion, diced **al**
½ Teaspoon Chili **al**
1 Rash Bacon, diced **ac, p**
1 Tablespoon Tomato Flesh, diced **al, p**
2 Cloves Garlic, crushed **ai, al**
2 Slices Bread **ac**
1 Teaspoon Thyme **al**
Olive Oil **mct, ai**
¼ Cabbage, sliced **al**
Season with Salt **al** and Cracked Black Pepper **ac**

Line a baking tray and brush with oil.

Peel skin from mushrooms, remove stems, and chop finely.

Heat oil in a frying pan; add onion, bacon, 1 clove crushed garlic, mushroom stems, thyme, and chili; cook until softened; remove and cool.

Blitz bread in a food processor.

In a bowl, combine bread and cooled mixture, lemon zest, tomato, and seasoning.

Place mushrooms on a tray and top with mixture.

Bake at 180° C for 20-30 minutes.

In a small frying pan, add olive oil, 1 clove crushed garlic, cabbage, and seasoning. Cook until wilted.

Serves 2

# PART 4

## "I Choose"

I wrote this chapter because one of the main problems with losing weight effectively and keeping it off is the psychological issues involved; emotional eating and other issues can be very complex. You need to start with a plan. That plan does not include a diet!

Diet at the front of this book stands for:

**D**igestion, **I**mmunity, **E**ducation, and **T**asty

A proper diet should ease digestion, boost immunity, and provide quality education, and most of all, the food should be tasty and easy to make.

The word "diet" in the Macquarie Dictionary states

1. particular selection of food especially prescribed to improve health or regulate weight
2. the usual or regular food a person eats most frequently
3. to follow a diet

The word "diet" from a thesaurus:

food
sustenance
tucker
count calories
fast
reduce
watch one's waistline

Let's look a little closer:

- "A particular selection of food … to improve health or regulate weight"; this has been outlined previously in this book with foods containing potassium, acids, alkalines, and medium chain triglycerides, foods which are free of sulphites, mineral salts, and trans fats.
- Eat fresh, unprocessed foods in season and in abundance. When I think of processed foods, I instantly think of road kill; this turns me off the idea of eating any of it. Processed foods are dead food. This book provides a repertoire of recipes to help get you started in cooking with fresh ingredients
- "The usual or regular food a person eats most frequently"; all of our recipes use everyday foods found in your local supermarket or grocery store. There are no ingredients listed where you need to track deep into the jungle to gather!
- "To follow a diet"; I encourage you to not follow any diet but choose to make a lifestyle change.
- Our recipes contain foods with sustenance, but without the need to count calories, you won't need to fast, but you will watch your clothes become looser.

The meaning of the word "diet" to me is:

- Starting something to stop; lifestyle change is an ongoing option for life.
- Lifetime memberships to set you up to fail, so you can keep coming back.
- 12-week program; a lifestyle change has no ending.
- Rapid weight loss; patience is the key to sustainability.

If you see any of above being advertised, run, walk fast, roll, drive, skip, jump, or even hop away as fast as possible. It is a marketing strategy to take your money and feed only your low self-esteem and lack of assertiveness. However, I have patients who are diehard fans of these places, so I work together with them. I ask the patient what foods they are to eat and then simply apply my rules of thumb.

## Rules of Thumb

No sulphites or mineral salts; keep a checklist handy.
No trans fats, check labels.
Eat medium chain triglycerides, healthy fats, listed earlier in this book.
Try to buy organic meats.
Use natural pot set yoghurt and add your own fruit.
Try to eat foods 80 percent alkaline and 20 percent acid.
Replace snack bars with whole nuts and raw coconut for snacks or use the snack option recipes in this book.

If I think of the word "diet," I think

- not much food to eat
- feeling hungry
- feeling resentful
- sacrificing
- no fun
- pressure from time limits and meeting expectations
- secretly knowing it won't last
- secretly knowing I will put any lost weight back on, if I lose it in the first place, and putting more weight will be harder to lose next time, so why bother?

I learned some interesting information from a UK documentary called *The Truth About Fat.*

People are eating more food today because it is more accessible; people don't understand body triggers, which tell them when to stop. Hormones will tell you when to eat, if you are feeling hungry, when to stop eating and when you are feeling full. Appetite hormones tend to head towards foods which are fatty, salty, or sugary, which lead to processed foods, which are triggered by stress and emotional eating.

Bad food is as addictive as alcohol and drugs; diets are about habits, not will power.

Patients were placed into three categories: hormonal, psychological, or genetic factors of being overweight.

Hormonal patients tend to feast; the hormone signal to stop eating is weaker, and once they start, they cannot stop. These patients should eat high protein and low GI foods: fish, chicken, slow carbohydrates, pasta, bulga wheat, lentils, basmati rice, beans, grains, cereals. These foods arrive later in the gut and release more full hormones; you will feel fuller 8 hours longer. No potatoes, bread, or other rice. Feasters should put on their plates ¼ protein, ¼ low GI carbohydrates, ½ vegetables, and dessert should be fruit. Whole foods fill the gut with no space for gas. If you cook all of your nightly food and blend it into a soup, it takes longer to digest and sends signals of fullness.

Psychological patients are emotional eaters and eat due to stress; they have a tendency to eat 4 times more sweets, nuts, and chips. These patients work better with support groups either face to face, online, or via email. This helps to boost their motivation to keep them going.

Genetic patients are constant cravers; genes disrupt the brain, saying fat stores need replenishing. These patients work better with eating well for five days and two days per week have no more than 800 calories; this shocks the body into burning fat. Best foods on the two days of 800 calories are meat, fish, eggs, and vegetables; no carbohydrates.

I think lipoedema comes under all of these umbrellas.

## Key Points to Consider

- It takes more than three months to establish good eating habits.
- Exercise should be introduced after three weeks; a pedometer is the best tool for counting steps and movement; increase exercise gradually, weekly after the first month.

- A loss of fluid is generally the first large amount of weight lost in the beginning.
- Thick soups last longer in the gut and are more filling.
- Start to change your reward methods; don't use processed foods.
- Get to know your digestion.
- Three-quarters of successful dieters eat breakfast and regular meals.
- Larger people have a higher metabolic rate; the more weight that is lost, the slower your metabolism will become.
- Eat sitting down and take your time, taking about 30 minutes; chop your food up, put your knife and fork down between bites, and if you need to use a spoon eat with a small spoon.
- Exercising on an exercise bike for thirty minutes burns two hundred calories. Going shopping with a basket, talking on the phone standing for thirty minutes, walking for thirty minutes, going up and down stairs all use 270 calories. The advice is to do everyday activities and keep moving.

Unwittingly, I adopted the majority of these techniques well before I watched them on this documentary.

## What I Do and Eat

It has taken me years to get and keep my weight off, but now I don't have to think about what I can eat and what I can't; it just comes naturally.

- My exercise regime consists of stretching exercises and constant movement throughout the day, with various activities.
- I changed my reward methods.
- I got to know my digestion and what foods upset it and also the lymphatic-friendly foods that work with me, not against me.
- I eat breakfast and regular meals throughout the day.
- I take the time to eat my food outdoors in the sunshine, without distraction, over thirty minutes.

- I put my knife and fork down in between bites and eat using a small spoon.
- I did learn to read labels and know what was in the food I was buying.
- I don't eat red meat (there is a reason for this, and I will talk about it later) or pork.
- I have no caffeine (because I like to rely on my own body's energy), no added salt, no added sugar, no foods containing sulphites, no mineral salts or trans fats, and very limited to no dairy (due to being lactose intolerant).

I don't eat red meat because of a condition called "mammalia." According to the Australasian Society of Clinical Immunology and Allergy (ASCIA), tick allergies, particularly to red meat and gelatin, are on the rise in Australia, along the Eastern Seaboard down to Victoria, but they can be found in other countries also. Patients can become anaphylactic after eating this food over many years; early warning symptoms include bloating, feeling nauseous, and experiencing diarrhoea just after eating it. This happened to me every time I ate red meat. I didn't want the Alpha-gal building up in my system over time for me to then become anaphylactic; it was becoming a real problem. I also found it hard to digest red meat and noticed it caused inflammation in my body, which makes my lipoedema worse. So I avoid it for those reasons also.

I am not a dietician or doctor, and any changes of diet or elimination of food groups should be fully investigated first.

I am in no way a psychologist either, but I have learned to turn my destructive food behaviour around to favour me instead of hurting me, and I wanted to share that information with you. If you are struggling with emotional eating, I would recommend consulting a psychologist for professional assistance.

I was an emotional eater and craved both sugary and salty foods, which most of us do. I know I was an emotional eater because whenever I was stressed, bored, peer pressured, or lonely, I would eat. I would eat anything and everything that I would desire. If I didn't know what I desired, then TV advertising would come and help me out with adverts of fast food and junk food, and then I would have my answer. I would happily drive down to the shop and buy it, eat it, and want more until I burst. Then the guilt kicked in. It's such a vicious cycle.

I felt fat, unhappy, and ashamed for letting myself do that over and over again and not having the strength to stop. I was suppressing my feelings and mood swings and filling the voids in my life with food. It was generally bad food. I was constantly being told by Doctors I was heading for a heart attack or stroke and quickly. I just kept changing doctors.

I have now learnt what triggers these cravings, and I deal with those issues first before turning to the food substitutes. I learnt to conquer this emotional rollercoaster myself, with the help of my husband, over many years, but looking back now in hindsight, I would recommend getting professional help to learn what your personal triggers are.

Back in the early days of my marriage (I have now been married for eighteen years), I was quite large, and in fact, I was obese, according to my Body Mass Index. I travelled away for my work, up to four months of the year, and I would get horribly lonely; the fact that I couldn't cook left me with one alternative: take-away. I ate a large variety from fried chicken, pizza, and pasta to burgers, and for dessert, ice cream and chocolate biscuits, all washed down with sweet drinks.

I would drink a full bottle of Cottee's Mix-up Drink every week, and I put sugar on and in everything. I ate a packet of Tim Tams nightly after consuming all the fried take-away food. I smoked around fifteen cigarettes per day and was on the contraceptive pill. I did no exercise, because I was too burnt out from working all the time.

When I got the guilts, I would eat some more and hoped that no one knew. I was only kidding myself. I now know this was due to having no assertiveness.

I needed to have assertiveness to learn how to cook healthy foods to put into my body and have the respect for myself that I deserved. I learnt to love myself instead of being destructive to my body.

Healthy foods will allow me to live a long, healthy life so I can effectively do what I have been sent here for: my life purpose. We are all sent here to leave our mark, our legacy, to make the world a better place for the next generation that comes through. You can't do that if you're too consumed with diets, counting calories, and restricting yourself, which leads to resentment of yourself and others. All of this is unhealthy.

When I returned home from my business trips and was reaching for the chocolate biscuits, ice cream, or potato chips, my husband would ask, "Do you really need that?" I was completely offended by this comment and would think to myself, *How could he say something like that to me?*

My reply was an abrupt, "Yes, I do." And he would simply say, "Alright then" and go about his business.

This went on for a couple of years until one day, I started to think to myself, *I'm not really hungry. I don't know why I want this; am I just bored and eating for the sake of it? Am I frustrated? Am I lonely? Am I stressed? I don't think so.*

I actually was very stressed and didn't realise it at the time, until one day I collapsed in a heap on the floor, rolled myself into the foetal position, and cried all day. I was severely burnt out and suffered from post-traumatic stress syndrome. I needed to change jobs and fast.

When I fell pregnant with my son, in 2002, I suddenly had someone else to focus on. I took a long time off from work, and this gave me the space I needed to concentrate on my health. I needed to make my plan.

I wrote down the following:

1. What I wanted out of my life
2. Who I wanted in my life

3. What work I wanted to do
4. Where I wanted to do it
5. The hours I wanted to work
6. How much money I wanted to earn
7. Where I wanted to live
8. What activities I enjoyed doing

A week after having Ben (by C section), I went in for another operation, to remove my gallbladder. I had 40 gallstones spilling out of my gallbladder and into my thoracic duct, heading for my liver. This wasn't good, and it was mainly due to the many years of my bad eating habits.

After my gallbladder was removed, I found that I simply couldn't eat any types of fatty foods or I would become quite ill and nauseous; that feeling sometimes lasted up to a week. It felt like continuous morning sickness all over again.

By remembering how I felt after eating that type of food, I started to avoid it. I used those memories to draw inspiration to stop my cravings, and I still do this every day.

Just as your body adjusts to digesting unhealthy foods and starts to send the signals for more fat, salt, and sugar, your body will adjust to digesting healthful foods. You will start to crave them, and you will begin to notice that if you eat something unhealthy, your body will let you know through diarrhoea, constipation, gas, bloating, reflux, and that feeling of nausea.

Every single day of my life, I make the choice of what I put in my mouth.

I could quite easily be lazy and buy something unhealthy. I have never encountered something packaged as completely healthy. I take ownership and control of the choices that I make because I have learnt to respect my body through assertiveness.

I choose to learn about and read food labels to know what chemicals are going into the foods I buy.

My son, Ben, has Tourette's syndrome, a neurological disorder, accompanied with Asperger's syndrome, which is on the autism spectrum.

I can certainly tell you that when he eats processed, chemically laden food, usually given to him by his obese, diabetic grandmother, his tics increase, he is hyperactive, he has trouble focusing, his attitude darkens, and he gets angry quickly.

We keep him eating mostly healthful foods and have learned to get around any peer pressure of not eating any junk food. We cook home-made hamburgers, pizza, Thai food, Chinese food, Mexican food, and fish 'n' chips. We offer him the Sunset Spritzer (recipe in this book) as a fizzy drink substitute. This keeps him happy and feeling like he fits in with the other kids.

I choose to put food items back on the shelf or take them back if they contain anything that I don't want.

I choose to ask the waitress in a restaurant how the food is prepared, where it is obtained from, and whether any mineral salts were used.

I choose not to be peer pressured if everyone else is having something junky.

I choose to learn the effects BPA plastics have on my body.

I choose to learn what synthetic hormones change in my body so I can make the choice in taking them or not, particularly due to having lipoedema.

I choose to reward myself in other ways than eating unhealthy foods:

- Family fun activities, paper aeroplane competitions, craft activities, colouring, and so on.
- Having a relaxing, quiet bath with candles, music, and bubbles.
- Watching the sunrise or sunset and counting how many colours I can see.
- Deep breathing: positive-in, negative-out.

- Using positive words like, "I am feeling happy, healthy, and energetic."
- Buying myself some fresh flowers.
- Going for a walk on the beach, in the bush, or just down the road.
- Watching an old (or new) movie.
- Buying a new flavoured herbal tea.
- Gardening.
- Putting together a home-made pamper package: facial, legs, hair colour, manicure or pedicure, self-massage.
- Doing jigsaw or crossword puzzles.
- Read a new (or old) book.
- Yoga and meditation.
- Playing with the dog.
- Cooking or making up a new recipe.
- Making some sandwiches and going on an unplanned picnic.
- Going to the fish market and seeing all the lovely fresh produce I can buy.
- Learning something new.
- Going to garage sales.
- Going for a drive in the car.
- Go for a swim in a pool or in the ocean.
- Spending quiet time with my husband
- Cooking with my son

***"These are just a few things that I do, when I want to do something nice for me."***

## Basic Health Tips

1. Air out your house every day; this will clear out any built-up stale air. Avoid using sprays. It is better to use pump bottles.
2. Hang clothes on the outside line to soak up the Vitamin D from the sun.
3. Try to eat your breakfast outside, watching the sunrise.
4. Processed foods have as much life force as road kill.

5. Have a repertoire of basic recipes; this makes for easy cooking without having to put too much time or thought into preparation.

6. Look for (or start up) a community vegetable or herb patch; I often see vegetable or herb patches on the council land out the front of the house. Make sure you check with your local council first.

7. If you have a large vegetable patch or fruit trees, put any excess fruit or vegetables out the front of your home in a box or crate with a "Free" sign for other people to take home. I used to get my lemons this way.

8. Try your hand at cooking parties or instant restaurants at home, with friends rotating around like they do on the reality TV shows.

9. Try to do your own housework; it will save money on cleaners and gym fees (because it is a better workout regime), and you have the reward of a clean home, which will win you many compliments.

10. Eat local produce in season; this will save money, and you can cut down on supplements because you will be getting all of your nutrients from your food.

11. Instead of expensive, coloured sports drinks, you can add a granule of rock salt or Himalayan salt to your water; this will provide your healthy mineral salts for you.

12. Swish and rinse your teeth and mouth after drinking lemon or eating food; this will assist in neutralising your mouth and clean your teeth, and it is an incentive to drink more water.

13. If you get dry eyes, particularly after a windy day, try a dampened, heated face cloth over your eyes, pressing lightly along the edges of your eyelashes; this will clear out the tear ducts and open the lymph vessels to assist in clearing away any dust which may be causing the dry eyes.

14. Drinking lemon in warm-water first thing in the morning cleans away any built-up bacteria on the tongue that has accumulated overnight, preventing you from swallowing it and potentially getting sick.

15. By drinking your tea or coffee at home, prior to going shopping, you are eliminating the urge to have one at the shop along with a cake of sorts, saving money and calories.

16. Ward off illness by:

a) Blowing your nose after you have had a shower or bath; the mucous will be softened at that point for easy blowing.

b) Syringe your sinuses; using tepid water with a pinch of salt, draw the water up the syringe. Lean forward over the sink with your head tilted to one side and squirt. Blow your nose. Repeat on the other side. You should feel the water going up and around and coming out the opposite side. If your nose is blocked, then you might want to try it a couple of times in the one session and every day until the blockage has ceased.

c) Nasal breathing or deep breathing; breathe in through the nose and push the stomach out, then breathe out through the mouth and pull the stomach in, holding for the count of three. Release. Start again. I do about five per day, long and slow; you can add the arms like doing a Mexican wave for added benefits, or hold the pelvic floor muscles for a count of three.

d) Gargling with warm water and salt if you feel a sore throat coming on.

e) Lemon in your water or in your salad dressing provides a good boost of Vitamin C.

17. Try to eliminate alcohol, caffeine, and sugar; use your own energy. You will realise how little energy you have at first, but by changing some habits and making time for you, then you will notice your energy coming back without the help of substances.

18. Pushing back cuticles on fingers and toes will often break the barrier between the skin and nail; this causes infection.

19. Receiving or performing manual lymph drainage on your face daily. I do this using my face cream twice a day; it will keep you looking younger because you are getting rid of built-up toxins from your face, caused by make-up and air pollution.

20. Addressing hydration, both internally and externally; drink water and apply a skin lotion (not one with petroleum, lanolin, or mineral oils, which suffocates the skin), for optimum skin care and cell functioning.

21. Dry brushing or light massage on the backs of the upper arms can improve a slow lymph flow (little pimples on the arm indicate this condition), by stimulating the lymph vessels to pump more.

## Discipline, Diligence, Commitment, and Continuity

Yes, it takes discipline, diligence, commitment, and continuity to achieve anything, but I can certainly tell you with complete certainty

### it pays off, in your favour.

You will feel happier, be healthier, and have a brighter outlook on life, with plenty of energy to fulfill it.

If you take a closer look at nature, everything is in perfect order and sync to keep everything in balance and flowing smoothly.

The sun rises and sets every day; the moon comes out at night with the stars and governs the tide patterns; we have four season, every year, without fail; and there is structure and balance in the food chain in order for everything to survive.

Our bodies are a perfect example of continuity. Our brain sends many automated messages to keep us running smoothly: our heart to beat, our eyes to blink, our lungs to breathe. Without this organisation and dedication to our body, none of this would happen, and we simply wouldn't be here.

If you look at successful people, they are organised and disciplined in order to achieve the goals they have set for themselves.

People in our armed forces are fully regimented in their organisation and use disciplinary skills for survival.

Governments on all levels have structure and routine, right down to having your garbage emptied on the same day every week.

Sports people on many levels are disciplined, with their training routines and eating patterns for optimal performance and many other professions have structure, organisation, discipline, diligence, commitment, and continuity to be successful.

This is what we crave in many circumstances to keep up with the challenges that face us on a daily basis. Having a routine of regular eating times, regular healthy foods, daily exercise, family time, and work time helps us cope when life throws us a curve ball, which it will. If we are presented with something out of our routine, we will know how to deal with it.

You don't need to have a lymphatic disorder to benefit from this book; you just have to have a lymphatic system. I ask you to be honest with yourself and to know that you are worth the time and effort to invest in your life.

Don't waste another minute. Go and get a fist full of life. It tastes great!

Just remember: "I choose."

With love and light.

Kristin

A special thank you to Talk Lipoedema Support Group USA www.facebook.com/talklipoedema.org for all their assistance

# Resources

www.foeldicollege.com

www.casleysmithinternational.org/#section3

www.vodderschool.com/emil_vodder_life_work_article

chiklyinstitute.com/Products/Silent-Waves

Joachim E. Zuther Lymphoedema Management The Comprehensive Guide for Practitioners 3rd Edition.

apal.org.au/wp-content/uploads/2013/07/Rowan-Berecry.pdf

kherbst.startlogic.com/4801.html

www.essense-of-life.com

www.health.qld.gov.au/nutrition/resources

livelovefruit.com

www.drweil.com/drw/u/ART02995/Dr-Weil-Anti-Inflammatory-Food-Pyramid

www.foodstandards.gov.au/consumer/additives/additiveoverview

J Neurosci. 2015 Feb 11;35(6):2485-91.

Inspiration is the major regulator of human CSF flow.

Dreha-Kulaczewski S1, Joseph AA2, Merboldt KD3, Ludwig HC4, Gärtner J5, Frahm J2.

Kristin Osborn's clinic is located in Newcastle NSW Australia
www.newlymphclinic.com.au

Printed in the United States
By Bookmasters